ON THE EVOLUTION OF CONSCIOUS SENSATION, CONSCIOUS IMAGINATION, AND CONSCIOUSNESS OF SELF

Robert G. Kunzendorf
University of Massachusetts Lowell

Imagery and Human Development Series
Series Editor: Anees A. Sheikh

Routledge
Taylor & Francis Group
LONDON AND NEW YORK

First published 2015 by Baywood Publishing Company, Inc.

Published 2017 by Routledge
2 Park Square, Milton Park, Abingdon, Oxon OX14 4RN
711 Third Avenue, New York, NY 10017, USA

Routledge is an imprint of the Taylor & Francis Group, an informa business

Library of Congress Catalog Number:
ISBN 13: 978-0-89503-901-9 (hbk)
ISBN 13: 978-0-89503-902-6 (pbk)

Library of Congress Cataloging-in-Publication Data

Kunzendorf, Robert G.
On the evolution of conscious sensation, conscious imagination, and consciousness of self / Robert G. Kunzendorf.
pages cm. -- (Imagery and human development series)
ISBN 978-0-89503-901-9 (cloth : alk. paper) -- ISBN 978-0-89503-902-6 (pbk. : alk. paper) -- ISBN 978-0-89503-903-3 (e-pub) -- ISBN 978-0-89503-904-0 (e-pdf)
1. Consciousness. 2. Imagery (Psychology) 3. Senses and sensation. 4. Self. I. Title.
BF311.K845 2015
153--dc23
2015016906

To Liz

Table of Contents

PREFACE

In Pursuit of Consciousness

> If man is to live, he must act; and, if he must act, he must govern his actions in accordance with conceptions of his own nature and of the world in which he is set, conceptions of whose validity he can have no absolute guarantee. . . . And of all conceptions, the conceptions of the nature of, and of the relations between, mind and body are those which in the long run affect most profoundly, and are of the first importance for, this guidance of conduct; for they must always exert a determining influence upon man's view of his place in the world, upon his prospects, his hopes, and his deepest purposes, and hence upon his conduct.
>
> —*Body and Mind: A History and a Defense of Animism*,
> William McDougall (1911, p. 87)

The present book reflects my 40-year quest to understand the subjective experiences of sensation and self and the general nature of their relationship to the brain. This quest commenced during my undergraduate years at Yale College, during the Vietnam War. In the course of those years, it became apparent to me that people who attributed consciousness to an immortal soul were less opposed to sending college graduates off to war, whereas people who attributed consciousness to brain activity alone were more resistant to putting anyone's brain or life at risk in Vietnam. On one side of this metaphysical divide were substance dualists whose belief in a conscious soul that survives bodily death was grounded in religious faith, and on the other side were materialists whose commitment to understanding conscious existence in purely physical terms was based on faith in the future of science. But to me, neither faith-based approach was satisfactory, given the solemn implications of this metaphysical divide for young men anticipating military conscription. Ultimately, an intellectual pathway leading out of this dilemma and toward testable theoretical solutions emerged when Wendell Garner, in one of his seminars at Yale, urged us not to let the status quo unduly constrain our psychological theories or our empirical predictions. Instead, he argued, we should start with a problem or a hypothesis that is deeply interesting—even the mind-body problem or a hypothesis concerning consciousness—and should proceed by logically deducing and empirically testing predictions that take us beyond the status quo.

Electing to take this pathway in as many consciousness-related directions as possible, I have devoted my postcollegiate years to the pursuit of hypotheses and discoveries that might clarify some of the relationships between consciousness and the physical world. During graduate school at the University of Virginia, I pursued a major in cognitive psychology and a minor in the mind-body problem, and with the guidance of my advisor, Arthur I. Schulman, I wrote and defended a doctoral dissertation entitled *Imagery and Consciousness: A Scientific Analysis of the Mind-Body Problem*. During my first few years at UMass Lowell in the early 1980s, I was trained to do psychophysiological research on consciousness by Mitchell Brigell at Northeastern University, and I was introduced to hypnosis research on mind-body issues by Theodore Barber at Cushing Hospital. In the late 1980s, I joined Ernest Hartmann, Robert H. Harrison, and Deirdre Barrett in a monthly research group on conscious dream images (i.e., consciously imaged sensations in the absence of self-consciousness). In the early 1990s, before pursuing clinically oriented research into absences of self-consciousness, I took graduate courses in clinical psychology at Boston University, and I completed a clinical externship in Cambridge Hospital's Behavioral Medicine Program, with guidance and support from the program's director, Deborah Hulihan. Throughout all of these years, I have had the good fortune of being able to disseminate my empirical discoveries and theoretical conclusions in archival publications, particularly those edited by Anees Sheikh, by Jerome L. Singer, and by James Honeycutt. And in pulling together the fruits of my varied pursuits and summarizing them in this book, I am grateful for the feedback that I have received from Eugene Bliss, whose broad knowledge and insightful thinking I truly value.

Substantively, my research on conscious sensation, conscious imagination, and self-consciousness has converged on a theoretical position that is partly dualistic and partly materialistic: *double-aspect materialism*, which posits that our nervous systems are composed not only of physical aspects but also of subjective aspects or conscious qualities that cannot be reduced to anything known to be "physical" in the third-person sense. The crux of this position is that some conscious qualities must in and of themselves have causal effects on bodily processes. Otherwise, all conscious qualities can be reduced to corresponding behaviors or corresponding neural aspects and can be eliminated from scientific discourse, as both the behaviorists and the eliminative materialists maintain. To date, however, compelling evidence for the causal efficacy of conscious qualities per se has not been forthcoming. So, in this book, I am pursuing causal efficacy from a new theoretical angle: I am hypothesizing that the causal effects of consciousness are manifested primarily during the *evolution* of neural structures and their subjective sensory qualities; and to support my hypothesizing, I am presenting both some newly discovered data and some newly discovered relationships among old data.

During my 40-year quest, many people have given me the assistance and encouragement that I needed in order to move forward and that I appreciate in looking back. I am especially grateful to Ahmed Abdelal, Lavy Abramovitch, Linda Albright, Donna Allen, Dave Ambrose, the late John Armington, the late Ted Barber, Deirdre Barrett, Sue McLaughlin Beltz, Shelley Berlin, Gina McGlinchey-Berroth, Trish Boisvert, the late Larry Bott, Mitch Brigell, Eugene Brooks, Cindy Brown, Glenn Bubley, Franz Buker, the late Bill Butler, Dan Capone, the late Mike Chapman, Michelle Chapwick, the late Veda Cobb-Stevens, Stuart Cohen, Paul Coppens, Amedeo D'Angiulli, Annette Davis, the late Jim Deese, Tom Dinsmore, Kevin Doherty, Len Dupille, Nicole Dwyer, the late Bob Eason, Bob Enik, Steven Flier, Michelle Foran, Debbie Friedman, Bob Gamache, Wendell Garner, Nate Garvin, Len Giambra, Reid Gray, Onur Güntürkün, Scott Hall and Claire Hoffman Hall, the late Bob Harrison, the late Ernie Hartman, Rick Harvey, Tom Hersey, Victor Hilts, Jim Honeycutt, Diane Hoyle, Deb Hulihan, Bob Innis, Mike Justice, Julie Karpen, Kim Reynolds Kelly, Eric Klinger, Keith Kluender, Jim Kostoulakos, Chris Krueger, Roberta Kunzendorf and the late "Zeke" Kunzendorf (my parents), Priscilla Lacourse, Dave Landrigan, the late Vija Lusebrink, Scott and Natallia Lyman, Steve Lynn, Elaine Major, Charlotte Mandell, Joan Maurer, Jack Mayer, Allyssa McCabe, Michelle McGlone, Marty Meehan, Jacquie Moloney, Lynn Montisanti, Cindy Moran, Steve Moses, Janet Paroskie, Rose Paton, Neal Peachey, Charlie Rader, the late Starling Reid, the late Zelma Ritvo and the late Martin Ritvo, Gene Rogers, Bob Sansom, Art Schulman, the late Eleanor Shalhoup, Anees Sheikh, Mitch Shuldman, Richard Siegel, Jan Sima, Jerry Singer, Chris Smith, Stu Smith, Evelyn Solomon, the late Nick Spanos, Boly Taing, David Thompson, Bob Tracy, Nicole Treantafel, Jim Veatch, Tristan Visconti, Ben Wallace, Carlene Carrabino Wentland, Jayne Wilson, Kara Young, and, above all, my wife Liz Ritvo.

CHAPTER 1

Theoretical Background and the Current Evolutionary Hypotheses

> There is a sense in which I share the underlying motivation of the reductionists—to see how a unified theory of consciousness and the brain might be logically possible. But whereas they wish essentially to bring the mind within the domain of physical science, I believe that to be impossible; rather, the methods of scientific description, analysis and explanation have to be extended to include the mind. . . . We should have in mind the ideal of an explanation of consciousness that shows it to be a necessary feature of certain biological systems—an explanation that allows us to see that such systems could not fail to be conscious. . . . I think it is inevitable that the pursuit of such an account will lead to an alteration of our conception of the physical world.
>
> —"What is the Mind-Body Problem?"
> Thomas Nagel (1993, pp. 6–7)

On sunny weekends when my wife and I go out for an afternoon walk, I look up at the sky, experience conscious sensations of blueness, and am self-conscious that *I am perceiving the blueness*. On dark nights when I dream about blue skies, I also experience conscious sensations of blueness, but throughout my subconsciously imaged dream, I am not self-conscious that *I am imaging the blueness*. Why do our brains represent sky as bluish sensations instead of reddish sensations or melodious sensations or no sensations at all? Indeed, why have conscious sensations of blueness evolved at all? And why do our brains generate sensations that are accompanied by self-consciousness when we are awake but are unaccompanied by self-consciousness when we are dreaming? That is, why has wakeful self-consciousness evolved?

In developing answers to these questions and related ones, I will be generating and testing evolutionary hypotheses that are derived from the psychophysical theories of the philosopher Gottfried Leibniz, the psychological scientists Gustav Fechner and Oswald Külpe, the clinical psychologist Morton Prince, and the neuropsychologist Charles Sherrington. Testing the *axiomatic value* of an evolutionary hypothesis or any other hypothesis is practically impossible, of course, as this requires that all alternative hypotheses be proven false. But as a scientist, I am primarily interested in testing the *discovery value* of hypotheses rather than their axiomatic value. Whereas the scientific theory of evolution has guided physical anthropologists to newly discovered data showing the anatomical relatedness of birds to bird-hipped dinosaurs and the genetic relatedness of human beings to chimpanzees, the religious notions of creationism and "intelligent design"[1*] have led us to no such undiscovered truths in anatomical or genetic data. And whereas scientific models of self-consciousness have guided psychologists to newly discovered data showing the relatedness of hallucinated imagination to dissociated perception, the religious notion of a soul has afforded us no such discovery value. Accordingly, this book's hypotheses regarding conscious sensation, conscious imagination, and self-consciousness are intended to lead us to previously undiscovered truths in new data and to previously undiscovered relationships among old data—truths and relationships that might also be explained by reformulating alternative theses after the fact, but that would never be uncovered by such theses in the first place. Bearing this intention in mind, let us proceed by focusing on the theoretical approaches from which the evolutionary hypotheses in this book are derived.

CONSCIOUS SENSATION: SUBSTANCE DUALISM VERSUS ASPECT DUALISM

Historically, the development of psychological science is rooted in Gottfried Leibniz's (1765/1896) theoretical challenge to Cartesian dualism. According to René Descartes' (1641/1988) dualism, a soul-like "subject of consciousness" or nonphysical "homunculus" is *conscious of* "objects of consciousness," all of which are physical in substance. For Descartes, even visually imagined "objects of consciousness" are physical in quality, and only "pure understanding" without any sensory qualities is substantively nonphysical.

> In the act of understanding the mind turns as it were towards itself, and contemplates one of the ideas contained in itself; in the act of imagining, it turns to the body, and contemplates something in it resembling an idea understood by the mind itself. (p. 36)

The Cartesian assumption that all "objects of consciousness" are physical is naïvely adopted by most practitioners of behavioral science, cognitive science, and neuroscience. In embracing the animal as a physical model of human behavior and eschewing introspective data within the human mind, the behavioral scientist B. F. Skinner (1974) argued that introspective observers of an external object like salt do not really "have a salty taste" but simply "taste salt" (p. 78). And in "consider[ing] events taking place in the private world within the skin," Skinner

*Endnotes begin on p. 83.

argued that "what is felt or introspectively observed is not some nonphysical world of consciousness, mind, or mental life but the observer's own body" (pp. 16–17). What or who then is the "subject of consciousness" that observes an "object of consciousness" such as salt or the body? In embracing the computer as a physical model of the human mind, the cognitive scientist Bernard Baars (1988) argued that nonconscious representations in the mind's computer-like memory become "conscious events [which] are *objectlike*" (p. 187) by "gain[ing] access to the global workspace" or working memory (p. 43). What or who is *conscious of* the objectlike events in the global workspace? In embracing the physical brain as a third-person starting point for modeling human consciousness, the neuroscientist Daniel Schacter (1989) argued that "for explicit remembering to occur, the output of declarative/episodic memory must be able to gain access to CAS [Conscious Awareness System]" (p. 366) and that "a posterior region of the cortex, critically involving the inferior parietal lobes, constitutes part of [the] system subserving conscious awareness [CAS]" (p. 370). Who or what then is *conscious of* the memories that "gain access" to the brain's parietal lobes? To the extent that the behavioral scientist, the cognitive scientist, and the neuroscientists reject the immaterial Cartesian soul, they must suppose that a *neural* "subject of consciousness" is somehow *conscious of* physical objects—a question-begging supposition that amounts to "Cartesian materialism" and as such is criticized by Daniel Dennett (1991), Susan Blackmore (2004), and Eugene Brooks (2004–2005).

Deeming it impossible for any physical or nonphysical entity to be *conscious of* anything outside itself, Gottfried Leibniz (1765/1896) reconceived the soul as a nonphysical "bundle of sensations" paralleling neural events in the brain and representing the physical world outside the brain. Accordingly, the soul is not *conscious of* any physical objects in the brain or any nonphysical entities in the mind. Rather, the soul is *composed of* conscious sensations, which, on Leibniz's account, are nonphysical in substance and are subjectively transformed in parallel with physical transformations in the nervous system. It is important to note that both Leibniz's psychophysical parallelism and Descartes' (1641/1988) subject-object metaphysics were conceptualized in the terms of *substance dualism*, which posits the existence of souls that are nonphysical in substance and objects that are physical in substance. Ultimately, the psychophysicist Gustav Fechner (1860/1966) reinterpreted Leibniz's psychophysical parallelism in the terms of *aspect dualism* or double-aspect materialism. Fechner maintained that conscious sensations are the *subjective aspects* or *subjective qualities* of particular neural states. Thus, the mind is not *conscious of* sensations; subjectively, the mind is its sensations, and physically, it is the nervous system with those subjective aspects.

The most compelling example of such a subjective quality or conscious sensation is the visual after-sensation. Certainly, the circular pink after-sensation that remains after staring at a green circle for 2 minutes is neither a pink object in the world outside the body nor an object in the gray matter of the brain, but is the *subjectively pinkish quality* of particular neurons in a particular state of excitation. Furthermore, Fechner (1860/1966) was correct to assume that after-sensations of this sort do not differ qualitatively from subjectively similar sensations that are immediately perceived, given Kunzendorf, Thompson, and Butler's (1995-1996) demonstration that the pink after-sensation following a green percept and the pink sensation in a pink percept are not distinguishable under experimentally controlled conditions.

Historically, the above-described movement away from Descartes' (1641/1988) subject/object dualism and toward Fechner's (1860/1966) psychophysical parallelism made psychological science possible. Cartesian dualism presupposed that physical "objects of consciousness" can be scientifically measured and studied, but that the immaterial and unextended "subject of consciousness" constituting the mind cannot. In contrast, Leibniz's (1765/1896) psychophysical parallelism implied that the "bundle of sensations" comprising the mind can be introspectively described. Plus, Fechner's psychophysics demonstrated that the subjective brightness of a visual sensation can be logarithmically related to the physical intensity of light stimulating that sensation, if the light's changing intensity is recorded every time the sensation becomes twice as bright or half as bright. Co-founding psychological science on Leibniz's and Fechner's groundwork, Wilhelm Wundt (1863/1894) introspectively described the mind's "bundle of sensations," and William James (1890) insightfully described the mind's "stream of consciousness." Neither Wundt nor James deemed it necessary to describe parallel brain events, given that one's knowledge of all physical events must be mediated by one's conscious sensations representing those events. Like Leibniz, Wundt advocated substance dualism and equated the soul with the "bundle of sensations" paralleling the brain. In contrast, James (1890, Vol. 1, p. 182) advocated "empirical parallelism" and argued that psychological scientists could and should ignore the metaphysical question of whether the mind's sensations constitute *subjective aspects* of the brain, as Fechner argued, or an *immaterial substance* paralleling the brain, as Leibniz argued.

The metaphysical question raised by Leibniz (1765/1896) and Fechner (1860/1966) was not ignored by 20th century philosophers, however. Mind-brain identity theorists like Herbert Feigl (1958), Stephen Pepper (1960), and John J. C. Smart (1959) asserted that the mind and the brain constitute a single physical entity that doesn't possess any nonphysical subjective qualities, but that presents as conscious sensations from a subjective or first-person *perspective* and as neural states from an objective or third-person *perspective*. By implication, then, it should be possible to predict this physical entity's objectively observable behaviors from its objectively knowable brain dynamics, without paying any attention to its corresponding sensations. It should be possible, in other words, to replace psychological science with behavioral neuroscience. Countering these reductionist implications of identity theory, the double-aspect materialist Thomas Nagel (1974) argued that the bat's sensations, whatever they may be like, cannot be reduced to or known from third-person observations of bat echolocation but can only be known as the subjective aspects of being a bat. And further countering the epiphenomenalist implications of any mind-to-brain reduction, Nagel (1993) argued that one reason why the brain's subjective aspects cannot be reduced to its physical aspects is because some of those subjective aspects can have causal effects on the brain's physical dynamics.

CURRENT HYPOTHESIS REGARDING THE EVOLUTION OF CONSCIOUS SENSATION

Following the lead of Nagel's (1993) aspect dualism, Chapter 2 explores the hypothesis that the painful subjective quality of the harm-sensing nociceptor was the first sensation to be naturally selected and that sensations of pain evolved into a variety of sensory qualities paralleling the variety of sensory transmitters that evolved from nociceptors. The nociceptor has the primitive physical quality of a free nerve ending, and its subjective quality of pain has the causal effect of reinforcing trial-and-error behaviors that promote damage-avoidance, healing, and hence, survival. Moreover, there are three variations of the nociceptor. The heat nociceptor, the pressure nociceptor, and the chemical nociceptor are innervated, respectively, by harmful heat, by harmful pressure, and by harmful chemicals. The evolutionary hypothesis to be developed and defended is: (a) that some heat nociceptors evolved into pain-free heat or temperature receptors paralleled by sensations of temperature, others into airborne/waterborne-heat or light receptors paralleled by visual sensations; (b) that some pressure nociceptors evolved into pain-free pressure or touch receptors paralleled by sensations of touch, others into airborne/waterborne-pressure or sound receptors paralleled by auditory sensations; and (c) that some chemical nociceptors evolved into pain-free chemical or taste receptors paralleled by sensations of taste, and others into airborne/waterborne-chemical or smell receptors paralleled by olfactory sensations. "The retina is thus a group of glorified 'warm-spots,' the cochlea a group of glorified 'touch-spots,'" as Sir Charles Sherrington (1911, p. 324) pointed out. But notably, as the sensations paralleling thermal, visual, tactile, auditory, gustatory, and olfactory receptors have evolved from the painful sensation paralleling a particular type of nociceptor, they have not retained the reinforcing quality or the survival value or the usefulness of the nociceptor's subjective quality of pain. As Susan Blackmore (2004) notes in her book's chapter on the Evolution of Consciousness, "Some useless traits survive because they are by-products of other traits that have been selected" (p. 146). And compared to pain, sensations of greenness and redness and saltiness and sourness are subjectively useless.

Some of the supporting evidence reviewed in Chapter 2 shows that simple mutations can transform a chemical nociceptor into a taste receptor, a pressure nociceptor into a touch receptor, and a heat nociceptor into a temperature receptor.

Other supporting evidence shows that the first primitive eye to evolve—the eyespot of the flatworm—functioned like an airborne heat nociceptor, not like an avian or mammalian eye capable of seeing visual structure. Chapter 2 concludes by considering evidence that the central nervous system (CNS) serves, physically, to process neural signals emanating from sensory transmitters and, subjectively, to generate "tacit knowledge" (Fodor, 1968) in relation to the transmitters' conscious sensations.

CONSCIOUS IMAGINATION: IMAGISTIC THOUGHTS VERSUS IMAGES CONSTRUCTED FROM IMAGELESS IDEAS

Historically, the psychological study of conscious imagination has been at the crossroads of different approaches to the relationship between the mental and the physical. Psychology's German co-founder Wilhelm Wundt (1863/1894) and his British student Edward Titchener (1909) deemed it scientifically sufficient to introspectively study one's own sensations, which can be consciously and directly experienced as such. For the purpose of describing and understanding one's own thoughts, therefore, they deemed it sufficient to study the "centrally excited sensations" or mental images, which, in their own experience, composed all thoughts. Furthermore, based on introspective comparisons of vivid images with similar percepts, Wundt and Titchener argued that imaged sensations and perceived sensations were not qualitatively different, as Danish psychologist Harold Høffding (1891/1896) also argued:

> How does the free flow of ideas come to be recognized by consciousness as distinct from the actual percepts? There is, indeed, as a rule a difference in the degree of strength of a memory-image and a percept; but this difference may be very small, and may even quite disappear. . . . No grounds are present for arranging the content of consciousness in two different spheres, in the world of possibility and imagination on one hand, and the world of reality and perception on the other. On the contrary, this contrast is discovered only through experiences in great measure bitter. We must often run our head against reality, before it becomes clear to us where its limits lie. (pp. 130–131)

Contrary to such argumentation, however, Kunzendorf (1980, 1985–1986a, 2000) has repeatedly found that sensations with a perceptual source are normally distinguished more quickly from equally vivid sensations of imaginal origin than from fainter sensations of imaginal origin. And based on such findings, Kunzendorf (1987–1988) has theorized that the greater number of "centrally excited" neural impulses behind mentally imaged sensations of greater vividness is physically detected more quickly by the brain's source-verification process and is subjectively paralleled more quickly by the sensationless knowledge that *one is imaging* (*rather than perceiving*). On a philosophical level, this theory that the source of sensations is verified neurally and known tacitly (i.e., sensationlessly) implies that, even though one's mind cannot be *conscious of* any physical object outside the body or inside, one's mind can *tacitly know* whether the conscious sensations composing its subjective aspects are imagined or perceived. Accordingly, when one perceives a human brain in the laboratory, one's sensations are accompanied by self-consciousness that *one is perceiving*, but when one images a Cartesian soul inside the pineal gland, one's sensations are accompanied by self-consciousness that *one is imaging.*

Oswald Külpe (1893/1895), founder of the Würzburg school of psychology, was the first psychologist to conclude that the mind's subjective aspects include not only perceived sensations and "centrally excited" or mental imaged sensations but also tacit or "imageless" thinking in relation to those sensations. Ultimately, Külpe's imagery research led him to suggest that visually imaged sensations are subjective qualities of the retina and are centrifugally constructed from "imageless" cognition in the central nervous system (CNS)—a suggestion consistent with this book's first hypothesis: that nociceptors and their subjective qualities of pain evolved into the other sensory receptors and their modality-specific qualities of sensation.

Külpe's (1893/1895) evidence for "centrally excited sensations" of perceptual vividness came not from first-person observations of his own mind but from third-person observations:

> Several trustworthy observers have stated that they are able to call up at will visual sensations of definite quality and of equal vividness with those of external perception. These visual qualities are as a rule quite clearly distinguishable from ordinary memorial images. And as in certain extreme cases they have been found to give rise to after-images, there can be absolutely no doubt that the peripheral organs are concerned in their origination. (pp. 434–435)

Similarly, Külpe's evidence for "imagless thought" came not from first-person observations but from third-person observations of an imageless thinker:

> I have made observations upon several persons with a view to determining their power of the recollection (reproduction) of colour tones. We sat in a darkened chamber, and I required my subjects to reproduce definite colours, which I named to them in any order: yellow, green, red, etc. In most cases the reproduction was effected with more or less vividness in some 10 Sec. But one observer was absolutely incapable of forming a sensory idea of any coloured objects. He saw nothing, in spite of all his efforts, and although plenty of time was allowed him. His visual perception was quite normal, and he stated that he had never had illusions. I had no opportunity of testing his auditory reproduction. The process of recognition, so far as I could discover, was entirely normal. Here then, we have a person who recollects and remembers without memory images, and has thoughts and ideas without images of imagination. (p. 176)

According to Karl Bühler (1907/1964), a member of Külpe's Würzburg school, such imageless thought tends to embody rules and relations that transcend any particular sensory experience, and thus, "consciousness of a rule is not the rule, but rather the state of affairs [the particular sensations] from which it might possibly be derived" (p. 163).

Külpe's (1893/1895) observation-based conclusion that vivid visual imagers construct visual sensations from their imageless visual thoughts, whereas imageless thinkers do not, has received support from over two dozen 20th century findings of no correlation between the vividness of people's visual imagery and the correctness of their visuo-spatial problem-solving (findings reviewed in Chapter 3) and has recently received support from Zeman et al.'s (2010) finding of normal visual thinking, albeit imageless thinking, in a man who, after an angioplasty-induced ischaemic event, lost his ability to construct visually imaged sensations. Still, even though Külpe's constructivist conclusion explains all the null correlations between image-vividness and problem solving, it begs the question why visually imaged sensations are ever constructed (much less constructed on the retina) if the vivid imagers who construct them don't benefit from them. Indeed, given early findings of no correlation between the subjectively reported experience of image vividness and the objectively measured quality of problem solving, the first behaviorist, John Watson (1913), deemed mental images to be epiphenomena that need not be studied by behavioral scientists. And given continued findings of no correlation throughout the 20th century, even the imagery researcher Stephen Kosslyn (1994) deemed the mental image to "refer to the internal representation that is used in information processing, not the experience itself" (p. 3).[2]

In some 21st century studies reviving and refining Külpe (1893/1895) and Bühler's (1964) viewpoint, however, more vivid imaging has been shown to correlate positively with faster learning of the rules of topological equivalence (Kunzendorf & Reynolds, 2004–2005), faster learning of the rules of bird's-eye perspective (Kunzendorf & Buker, 2008–2009; Kunzendorf, Lyman, Sousa, & Hilly, 2012–2013), and faster learning of the rules of an artificial grammar (Kunzendorf et al., 2012–2013)—when research participants are instructed to figure out the actual rules by constructing mental images from their hypothesized rules. In other words, vivid imagers can construct "centrally excited sensations" from "imageless rules" that are under development, in order to test rule-derived sensations against remembered or perceived ones and to refine rules in need of further development. Thus, we should not be surprised that the individuals exhibiting the greatest vividness on self-report and objective measures of visual imagery are the child and the visual artist, both of whom are still developing their "imageless" visuo-spatial rules (Howie, Markham, & Kleitman, 2006; Kunzendorf, 1989; Kunzendorf, Justice, & Capone, 1997; Leonard & Lindauer, 1973; Lindauer, 1977; Morrison & Wallace, 2001; Pérez-Fabello & Campos, 2007).

Interestingly, based on his own observation-based conclusions (as described above) and on anatomical observations by Ramon y Cajal (1888, 1889), Külpe

(1893/1895) propounded the metaphysical thesis that, from "imageless" thoughts and memories in the central nervous system (CNS), vivid visual imagers construct "centrally excited sensations" and, in parallel, innervate physical aspects of the retina; whereas imageless thinkers do not centrifugally innervate their retinas and do not, in parallel, construct visually imaged sensations. This thesis not only serves as a corollary to the current hypothesis that subjectively painful qualities of the heat nociceptor evolved into visual qualities of the retina but also serves to resolve Roger Sperry's (1976) problem of being unable "to find a distinction between [CNS] events that involve consciousness and those that lack consciousness" (p. 166). Indeed, Külpe (1893/1895) framed his metaphysical thesis in terms of this latter problem:

> The latest anatomical investigations show that the sensory centres are very uniform in structure; whereas the peripheral sense organs present obvious differences, which are plainly of importance for differences in the conscious processes which they mediate. If we continue to speak of specific energies, we must consequently localize them in the peripheral sense organs. Look at the two higher senses, and see how admirably the structure of the eye is adapted to its spatial duty, and the structure of the ear to its qualitative function! The specific significance of the external organs is also evidenced by the fact that their removal absolutely prevents the appearance of sensible qualities in consciousness, while extirpation of the corresponding central organs may to a certain extent be compensated by the activity of others. . . . There is, however, one recent discovery of which mention must be made, as it seems to throw light upon many points of difficulty in the theory of sensation—the discovery of sensory nerve fibres with centrifugal conduction. These have been carefully examined in the case of the optic nerve, and may be presumed to exist in all the sensory nerve trunks. Side by side with the sensory fibres, in the usual meaning of the term, which take their origin in the peripheral organs and terminate in the brain, there will then be another set of sensory fibres, originating in the brain and ending in the sense-organ. . . . Lastly, we may imagine that the "centrally excited" sensations—memorial images, as they have also been very inappropriately named—are at least in many instances correlated with a co-excitation of the peripheral organs. (pp. 84–85)

Recent empirical findings associating mentally imaged sensations with centrifugally innervated receptors in the peripheral nervous system (PNS) will be reviewed in Chapter 3.

It is important to note that, whereas *fin-de-siècle* scientists like Oswald Külpe (1893/1895) and Sir Charles Sherrington (1911) inferred that conscious sensations are the subjective aspects of sensory receptors and that sensationless cognitions are the subjective aspects of cortical areas, 20th century Cartesian materialists like Francis Crick (1994) and Bela Julesz (1971) inferred that conscious sensations are the subjective aspects of cortical areas. This important inferential difference is perhaps best exemplified by the differing interpretations that Sherrington and Julesz put forth regarding the "singleness" or "Cyclopean nature" of the binocular percept.

Sherrington (1911) interpreted binocular experience in terms of "sensations generated in the two retinae" (p. 382):

> During binocular regard of an objective image each uniocular mechanism develops independently a sensual image of considerable completeness. The singleness of the binocular perception . . . is therefore the product of a synthesis that works with already elaborated sensations contemporaneously proceeding. (pp. 382–383)

> The convergence of nerve-paths from the right and left retinae respectively toward one cerebral region is significant of union for coordination of motor reaction rather than for synthesis of sensation. (p. 354)

Consistent with Sherrington's interpretation, stereoscopic studies confirm that, when half of a figure's structure is visible within one eye's sensations and the other half of the figure's structure is visible within the other eye's sensations, selective attention to the figure's structure across the two eyes' sensations produces the illusory experience of fused sensations (Kovács, Papathomas, Yang, & Fehér, 1996; Kunzendorf, 2009). Interestingly, the reason why one is not aware of the eyes' separate sensations is because CNS calculations lead to imageless knowledge about which side of the visual field a given monocular sensation comes from, not which eye it comes from (Kunzendorf, Butler, & Pearson, 1988; Ono & Barbeito, 1985). The reader can introspectively appreciate the binocular illusion of "fused sensations" without a stereoscope by doing the exercise in Appendix A and abstracting the binocularly structured diamond, then the binocularly structured heart, from the two eyes' sensations.

In opposition to Sherrington (1911), Julesz (1971) maintains that conscious sensations emerge in the cortex as part of a "cyclopean" percept, which is generated after sensationless information is abstracted from each eye and is unconsciously evaluated for its binocular disparities. In research employing random-dot stereograms in which no shape is monocularly perceptible, Julesz finds that, nevertheless, a square-shaped pattern of binocularly displaced dots is stereoscopically perceived as closer depthwise than the background pattern of binocularly corresponding dots. The issue is whether a "cyclopean" three-dimensional model of a dotted square above a dotted background is consciously generated in cortical area V3, as Julesz suggests, or whether randomly distributed dots in the left eye and systematically displaced sensations in the right eye are contemporaneously conscious while a square-shaped pattern of closer dots is cortically calculated and imagelessly inferred from the two eyes' sensations, as Sherrington suggests—and as Kunzendorf and Butler (1992) demonstrate to be the case.

In purely neural terms, retinal stimulation leads to the calculation of edges and their orientations in cortical area V1, then to the calculation of retinal disparities in cortical area V2, the computation of three-dimensional forms in cortical area V3, the computation of color constancies in cortical area V4,[3] and the calculation of direction of movement and rate of movement in cortical area V5. Given that the color and form of an object reflecting light onto the retina are neurally represented as separate features in separate areas of the cortex, Crick (1994) suggests that the object's color features and shape features must be *bound together* by cortical oscillations of 40 Hertz in order to bring the whole object into the "'spotlight' of visual attention" (p. 62) or "visual awareness" (p. 68). Of course, Crick's suggestion raises the specter of a Cartesian "subject of consciousness," a nonphysical or physical subject that is "aware of" the oscillation-*bound* object being brought into the "spotlight of visual attention."

Unlike Crick (1994), Külpe (1895) suggests that an object reflecting light onto the eye stimulates *retinal sensations*, which are accompanied neurally by many CNS calculations and subjectively by many "imageless thoughts" about the color constancy, shape constancy, and size constancy of the sensations representing the object. So for instance, as I sit at my desk and look down at my hands and shoes, it not only is the case that the brownish sensations composing my left shoe are darker than the brownish sensations composing right shoe (in accord with the third endnote's discussion of color constancy) but also is the case that the extension or length of my left shoe's sensations is phenomenally shorter than the introspected extension of my left hand's sensations. Accompanying my left shoe's shorter set of darker brown sensations, however, are *imageless* or *sensationless* inferences that my left shoe is farther away but not shorter than my left hand and is not browner than my right shoe. Furthermore, to the extent that the brown sensations themselves are the subjective qualities of adjacent retinal cells, rather than disparate cortical neurons, they need not in any additional way be *subjectively bound* to each other (or to any *sensationless* cortical inferences in relation to them). In other words, Crick's "binding problem" is a pseudo-problem from the standpoint of Külpe (1895) and Sherrington's (1911) conclusions that visual sensations are subjective qualities of the retina.

Obviously, Külpe (1895) and Sherrington's (1911) conclusions are consistent with this chapter's first hypothesis regarding the evolution of visual sensations in the retina from painful sensations in the heat nociceptor. Let us now consider the second hypothesis, regarding the evolution of visual images or "centrally excited" sensations at the retinal level.

CURRENT HYPOTHESIS REGARDING THE EVOLUTION OF CONSCIOUS IMAGINATION

Following the lead of Külpe's (1895) constructivist theory of mental imaging, Chapter 3 explores the hypothesis that the rule-developing and image-constructing brain of warm-blooded animals evolved from the past-association-bound and unimaginative brain of cold-blooded animals. This psychophysiological difference between warm- and cold-blooded animals points to one of the rare discontinuities in evolutionary history. As psychological evidence reviewed in Chapter 3 indicates, only warm-blood animals exhibit *rapid eye movement* during sleep—*(REM)*, which parallels the construction of dream images in primates; and as physiological evidence is associated with the construction of dream images in humans—and as physiological evidence reviewed in Chapter 3 indicates, all mammals and birds exhibit "log brain weight to log body weight" ratios that are a quantum leap higher than the ratios exhibited by all reptiles and all other cold-blooded vertebrates. Other evidence reviewed in Chapter 3 documents the centrifugal innervation of sensory transmitters during vivid imaging, including dream imaging, the central innervation of mammalian prefrontal cortex and avian nidopallium caudolaterale during imageless rule-governed reasoning, and the innervation of imageless reasoning and vivid imaging during the hypothesizing and testing of new generative rules.

CONSCIOUSNESS OF SELF: "SUBJECT OF CONSCIOUSNESS" VERSUS ILLUSION OF "SELF AS SUBJECT"

When Gottfried Leibniz (1765/1896) posited that everyone's mind is a bundle of sensations paralleling physical events in one's nervous system, he also posited that one's sensations can arise with or without self-consciousness that *one is having them*. The latter philosophical position was a radical departure from the Cartesian position, which is best expressed by Charles Campbell (1957): "In self-consciousness, the subject of which we are conscious is a subject which in some sense *has*, not *is*, its different experiences, and is identical with itself in its different experiences" (p. 81). For the 19th century thinkers who built the science of psychology on Leibniz's (1896) philosophical foundations, self-consciousness was the illusion of "having" sensations, and it accompanied sensations only some of the time. In accounting for this illusion, Oswald Külpe (1893/1895) identified self-consciousness both with sensations of the bodily self and with imageless concepts of the psychological self:

> The development of *self-consciousness* has . . . a sensible root, in the visual or tactual demarcation of the subject's own body from the external world. . . . The language of daily life, and a whole number of pathological derangements of self-consciousness, furnish conclusive evidence that the visual and tactual idea of the body forms one of the most essential constituents in the idea of the self. It is not the sole constituent, of course: there is a mental content besides the sensible. The mental content varies in character and importance with the course of individual development, being largely determined by the scientific, moral and religious beliefs of the subject. (p. 449)

As per William James' (1890) theoretical dissection of self-awareness, however, Külpe (1895) accounted only for "me-ness"—the subjective experience of "self as object," either a mutable sensory object or a mutable conceptual object—and did not account for "I-ness"—the subjective experience of "self as subject," an unchanging and illusory subject to which one's sensations seem to belong. Indeed, by James' theoretical analysis, most 20th century studies of self-awareness—studies of deficient self-recognition in the autistic child (Ferrari & Matthews, 1983; Kunzendorf, McLaughlin-Beltz, & Tymowicz, 1991–1992; Spiker & Ricks, 1984), studies of self-dissociated amnesia in the hypnotized adult (Kihlstrom & Cantor, 1984; Kunzendorf, 1989–1990), studies of self-identification in the "split brain" patient's minor hemisphere (Sperry, Zaidel, & Zaidel, 1979)—have accounted only for the "self as object," not for the "self as subject."

James (1890) identified the illusory experience of "self as subject" with the imageless feeling of familiarity, which accompanies current sensations that have previously been experienced and which implies that those sensations belong to the same self who originally experienced them. In proposing an alternative to James' theory of I-ness, Kunzendorf (1987–1988, 2000, 2010) has identified the illusory experience of "self as subject" with the CNS verification of a sensation's central (or peripheral) source, in parallel with the tacit knowledge that *one is imaging (or perceiving) the sensation.* According to Kunzendorf, the Cartesian illusion that *one is "having" sensations* is simply the generic version of self-conscious knowledge that *one is imaging sensations* or self-conscious knowledge that *one is perceiving sensations.*

Kunzendorf's (2000, 2010) source-verification theory of self-consciousness, following the lead of Leibniz's (1896) theoretical approach, accounts for abnormal sensory experiences without self-consciousness as well. Thus, as Chapter 4 will show, in abnormal phenomena like subliminal percepts and dissociated percepts, one's sensations are not tacitly accompanied by self-consciousness that *one is perceiving,* and in abnormal phenomena like dream images and hallucinatory images, one's sensations are not tacitly accompanied by self-consciousness that *one is imaging.*[4] Source-verification theory's approach to conscious sensation *with* or *without* the illusion of "self as subject," accordingly, represents Kunzendorf's integration of Gustav Fechner's (1860/1966) psychophysical interpretation of Leibniz (1896) and Morton Prince's (1910, 1921, 1925) clinical interpretation of Leibniz, both of which merit extended discussion.

As the historian of psychology Edwin Boring (1929) notes, the first scientific support for Leibniz's (1896) position that conscious sensations can occur with or without self-consciousness that *one is perceiving them* came from Gustav Fechner's (1860/1966) psychophysical equation: $S = k \log R$, as graphed in Figure 1. In this equation, the variable S is a sensation's subjective magnitude (e.g., its brightness or loudness) measured in "jnd" units, integer units defining a "just noticeable difference" in magnitude between $S = 0$ and $S = 1$, a "jnd"

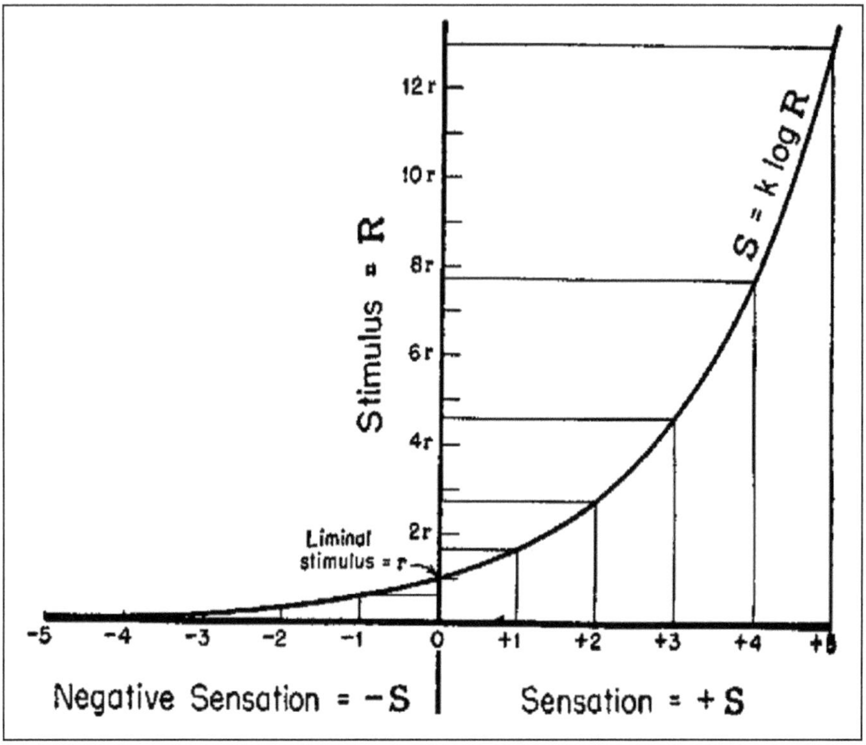

Figure 1. Fechner's psycholophysical equation: $S = k \log R$, where S is a sensations's subjective magnitude measured in units of *jnd* (units defined by the differential thresholds or *just noticeable differences* between subjective magnitudes), R is a stimulus's physical intensity measured in units of *limen* (a unit defined by the physical difference between zero intensity and the intensity at absolute threshold), and k is Weber's constant. As subjective magnitude increases arithmetically, physical intensity increases geometrically, resulting in a logarithmic function, where stimuli with intensities below one limen (the absolute threshold for self-conscious apperception) produce *negative sensations* or "subliminal" sensations. Adapted from *A History of Experimental Psychology* (Boring, 1929).

between $S = 1$ and $S = 2$, and so on. By definition, $S = 0$ is the "absolute threshold" at which a sensation of decreasing magnitude is no longer accompanied by self-consciousness that *one is perceiving it.* The variable R is a stimulus' physical intensity (e.g., its luminance or sound pressure level) measured in "limen" units, where 1 "limen" is the difference between zero intensity and the intensity at the absolute threshold. By definition, a stimulus is "subliminal" when $0 < R < 1$. Finally, the constant k is Weber's fraction $(\Delta R/R)$, a modality-specific fraction specifying the *relative change in stimulus intensity* that yields a "just noticeable difference" in sensory magnitude. Fechner's equation is historically important because, when $0 < R < 1$, mathematically, $S < 0$. And for Fechner, these negative sensations proved Leibniz was correct that self-consciousness can sometimes be negated while conscious sensations are being perceived. Leibniz's argument for the existence of "petites perceptions" without self-consciousness that *one is perceiving them* was thus transformed into Fechner's psychophysical equation demonstrating the presence of negative sensations during subliminal stimulation.[5]

The vast majority of psychologists no longer understand that "subliminal" means "below the absolute threshold for self-conscious apperception"—not since the computer metaphor for mind became psychology's *Zeitgeist* during the last quarter of the 20th century. Exemplifying this conceptual shift, the first chapter of Norman Dixon's (1971) book *Subliminal Perception* contains a discussion of Leibniz's work, whereas the first chapter of Dixon's (1981) book *Preconscious Processing* omits Leibniz altogether and intromits a flowchart that begins with a perceptual stimulus, progresses through a series of unconscious computer-like processes, and ends with a "conscious experience" (p. 6). Conceptually, inasmuch as the computer metaphor reduces all sensory and perceptual processes to unconscious computer-like processes, it only permits sensations to be epiphenomena at the late end of CNS processing and does not permit sensations to be subjective aspects of the sensory transmitters or the subcortical nuclei or the early cortical regions. But consistent with Kunzendorf's (1987–1988) reinterpretation of Fechner (1860/1966) in source-verification terms, several studies show that subliminally stimulated percepts are not sensationless entities, but are "subconscious sensations" devoid of any self-consciousness that *one is perceiving them* and, as such, are easily confused with mentally imaged sensations (Kunzendorf, 1984–1985; Kunzendorf & Butler, 1992; Kunzendorf & McGlinchey-Berroth, 1997–1998).

By the end of the 19th century, psychological study of the "subconscious sensation" unaccompanied by self-consciousness had undergone a paradigmatic shift, from the psychophysical phenomenon of subliminally stimulated perception to the clinical phenomenon of multiple personality. Cartesian dualism held that the "subject of consciousness" was an indivisible soul-like substance, but William James' (1890) memory-based explanation for an illusory "self as subject" implied that dissociated memories within a single person should give rise to the illusion of multiple "subjects of consciousness" within that person. In James' *1896 Lowell Lectures* (Taylor, 1984), he explained how some psychiatric patients with multiple personality disorder (MPD) have self-conscious personalities that contemporaneously emerge when one personality says one thing while another "automatically writes" something else, on account of memory systems that are neurologically dissociated but temporally overlapping. Other MPD patients have self-conscious personalities that emerge one at a time, on account of dissociated memory systems that emerge individually during different temporal segments of the waking state. Alternative selves may even arise in normal persons, during their dream life, if their nighttime memories are sufficiently dissociated from their daytime memories.

Morton Prince (1925) accepted James' (1890) theoretical distinction between the self-concept or the "self as object" and self-consciousness or "self as subject"; but based on clinical observation, Prince equated multiple personality with more than one "self as object," not with more than one "self as subject." Accordingly, Prince took issue with James' thesis that the contemporaneous activation of dissociated memory systems can give rise to more than one *self-conscious* personality at any given time:

> A plurality of coexisting selves is theoretically possible, particularly as we know that in the complex conditions of so-called multiple personality, dual (or more) selves occur, but . . . the empirical evidence entirely denies self-awareness to such conscious experiences. The introspective testimony of my dissociated subjects, who, in [the hypnotic] condition recalled vividly and precisely these subconscious experiences [of dissociated but coexistent personalities], has been unanimous that these experiences were without self-consciousness. (p. 182)

In his treatise on multiple personality, Prince (1921) described how a non-integrated personality unaccompanied by self-consciousness emerges into coexistence with the dominant personality shortly before self-consciousness shifts over to accompany the nonintegrated personality's fantasies and feelings instead of the fantasies and feelings of the dominant self-concept. And with regard to normal dreaming, Prince acknowledged that some dreamed sensations evoke a dissociated feeling of familiarity and hence a dissociated concept of self, but he also recognized that the dream's conscious sensations normally remain *subconscious*—unaccompanied by any self-consciousness that *one is imaging or dreaming*—until the dawn of wakefulness.

Prince's (1921) clinical approach to subconsciousness stands in contrast to Freud's clinical approach to unconsciousness. Instead of embracing Leibniz's (1896) psychophysical parallelism, Freud (1924) embraced the Cartesian assumption that the mind's contents and excitations are nothing more than unconscious objects, unless a "subject of consciousness" becomes *conscious of* them:

> The unconscious system may therefore be compared to a large ante-room, in which the various mental excitations are crowding upon one another, like individual beings. Adjoining this is a second, smaller apartment, a sort of reception-room, in which consciousness resides. But on the threshold between the two there stands a personage with the office of door-keeper, who examines the various mental excitations, censors them, and denies them admittance to the reception-room when he disapproves of them. . . . The excitations in the unconscious, in the ante-chamber, are not visible to consciousness

> which is of course in the other room, so to begin with they remain unconscious. When they have pressed forward to the threshold and been turned back by the door-keeper, they are "*incapable of becoming conscious*"; we call them then *repressed* . . . I should like to assure you that these crude hypotheses, the two chambers, the door-keeper on the threshold between the two, and consciousness as a spectator at the end of the second room, must indicate an extensive approximation to the actual reality. (pp. 305–306)

As Greenwald (1988) has noted, Freud (1924) actually posits two Cartesian subjects at two different locations in the mind—in the smaller reception-room, the "subject of consciousness" who is identified with self or ego, and on the threshold between rooms, the doorkeeper who, in order to repress certain objects, must first become aware of them. For Prince (1921), universal Freudian complexes are not repressed by a Cartesian gatekeeper, confined to the realm of unconscious objects and denied access to a Cartesian "subject of consciousness." Rather, for Prince, traumatic percepts and images are experienced as *subconscious* sensations, which are conscious and psychologically painful but, for the purpose of defending against such pain, are dissociated from self-consciousness. In Chapter 4, Prince's theoretical approach to the dissociation of self-consciousness from conscious sensations will be refined and reinterpreted in accordance with Kunzendorf's source-verification thesis, and research supporting this source-verification refinement will be reviewed.

CURRENT HYPOTHESIS REGARDING THE EVOLUTION OF SELF-CONSCIOUSNESS

In pursuance of Kunzendorf's thesis that self-consciousness serves to discriminate perceived sensations from vividly imaged sensations (of the sort that youngsters construct to test their developing rules), Chapter 4 explores the corollary thesis that self-conscious imagery-verification tends to evolve in those warm-blooded species whose maturing minds spend at least 2 years constructing vivid test imagery from newly hypothesized rules and whose survival prospects during those early years benefit from such imagery verification. Studies reviewed in Chapter 4 indicate that human source-verification processes are present during early childhood, are paralleled by the self-conscious experience of "self as subject" and are necessary for self-conceptions of "self as object" to develop. Additional studies indicate that such conceptions of "self as object" exist only in humans, chimpanzees, orangutans, gorillas, bonobos, elephants, dolphins, whales, crows, magpies, and parrots, all of whom require 2 or more years to mature into adult animals with fully developed cortexes and fully tested generative rules. Finally, after reviewing human research on individual differences in self-consciousness that *one is imaging* (*or perceiving*), Chapter 4 raises questions regarding future directions in human evolution.

EPILOGUE: SELF-CORRECTIVE TRENDS IN THE EVOLUTION OF CONSCIOUSNESS

The three hypotheses outlined above are logically independent with regard to their discovery value. But if all three hypotheses should be proven by the following three chapters to have such value, then the self-corrective pruning process that Darwin (1859) called "evolution" is itself in the process of being pruned by the evolution of mind.

Abstractly considered, the evolutionary processes of random mutation and natural selection have been functioning as a biological form of self-correction, but considered from the standpoint of any individual whose history of mutations has happened to reduce fitness for survival, random mutation and natural selection are cruel processes. However, as the peripheral nervous system's free nerve endings have evolved into heat and pressure and chemical nociceptors, the painful sensations paralleling nociceptor activation have motivated individual organisms in the animal kingdom to take self-corrective actions before damage of an objective form crueler than subjective pain takes its toll. Furthermore, as the central nervous system has evolved both the cognitive ability to generate hypothetical rules and the imaginal ability to anticipate their implications, an even less painful process of self-correction has arisen in warm-blooded animals. Finally, the natural selection of self-conscious reality-testing has served to correct for the fact that, without self-consciousness, the slow-developing children of certain warm-blooded animals do not know with any certainty whether their sensations are imagined or perceived.

We can only hypothesize and imagine what our descendants' self-corrective mental processes might be like 1,000 to 10,000 generations from now. But surely any descendents who survive and flourish in the distant future will have continued to evolve in a direction that has been influenced by the subjective and objective aspects of their self-corrective minds.

CHAPTER 2

The Evolution of Conscious Sensation

> Let us first be clear about where the problem of consciousness arises. It is sometimes mistakenly believed that this is at the point in a chain of behaviour (or in the evolution of behaviour) at which the most natural language to use employs the vocabulary of goals, intentions, etc. But there is no reason to suppose that a language in terms of goals and intentions implies the existence of conscious experiences in the behaving system. There are many ways in which one can design machines or programme computers so that they display goal-directed behaviours (i.e., so that they have "intentions"). But we have no reason to suppose (given our present absence of a suitable theory to guide us) that in so doing we are in some way "wiring in" consciousness. The problem of consciousness arises at a simpler stage in the business of machine construction than the stage at which it is necessary to build in goal-directed behaviour: it arises at the point of sensation.
>
> —"The Mind-Brain Identity Theory as a Scientific Hypothesis," Jeffrey A. Gray (1970, p. 251)

According to the hypothesis explored in this chapter, the evolution of conscious sensation started with the most primitive sensory receptors—the unmyelinated, high threshold, free nerve endings known as heat nociceptors, pressure nociceptors, and chemical nociceptors, which, when innervated by harmful heat or harmful pressure or harmful chemicals, manifest the irreducible subjective quality of pain. Throughout the course of evolutionary history, on this account, some heat nociceptors evolved into temperature receptors manifesting subjective qualities of pain-free heat, and others evolved into retinal receptors that respond to airborne or waterborne heat (i.e., light) and that manifest subjective qualities like visual brightness. Similarly, some pressure nociceptors evolved into touch receptors possessing subjective qualities of pain-free pressure, and others evolved into cochlear receptors that are responsive to airborne or waterborne pressure (i.e., sound) and that are paralleled by subjective qualities like auditory loudness. And likewise, some chemical nociceptors evolved into gustatory chemical receptors with pain-free qualities of taste, and others evolved into olfactory receptors that respond to airborne chemicals and manifest subjective qualities of smell. Consideration of this evolutionary history must begin, therefore, with consideration of the subjective quality of pain.

THE NATURAL SELECTION OF SUBJECTIVELY PAINFUL SENSATIONS

As Nagasako, Oaklander, and Dworkin (2003) note, "The sensation of pain protects humans (and other species) from the tissue-damaging effects of dangerous stimuli, and appears to be critical for survival of the organism" (p. 213). But as the following discussion shows, an organism in which subjectively painful sensation arises also needs a nervous system that can evaluate pain and can generate trial-and-error responses to it in order for the subjective quality of pain to have a causal effect on survival. Indeed, because pain is private, a young organism cannot simply be taught its father's standards for evaluating gradations of pain or for responding differently to different gradations. Rather, a young organism must evaluate its painful sensations according to its own privately defined gradations of tolerable and intolerable pain. And when a young organism deems pain to be intolerable, it must generate trial-and-error responses until it generates a response that either defies intolerable pain or reduces such pain to the organism's privately defined level of tolerability. (The author is well acquainted with young people's evaluations and responses, because his younger daughter always evaluated pain on a binary scale—"it still hurts" or "it's gone"; and unlike his older daughter, she always responded by defying her pain and engaging in the task at hand.)

One of two critical points to be emphasized here is that the subjective aspect of nociceptive innervation—the subjective quality itself—can be evaluated, and responded to, by an organism's nervous system. Let us consider how we judge and respond to our visual sensations, in order to fully appreciate this important point. The subjective aspects, as opposed to physical aspects, of my visual system are visual sensations that, in principle, I could communicate directly through a pictorial representation or indirectly through a verbal description or abstractly through an evaluative rating. And following the trial-and-error development of any one of these communication skills, I could generate a picture or description or evaluation of the bundle of visual sensations that constitute my conscious mind at a given moment. One of the notable differences between visual sensations and painful sensations is that I can give my daughters corrective feedback if they paint or describe or rate the sensations composing a publicly observable beet as *blue-green* rather than *red*, whereas I cannot unequivocally correct their descriptions or ratings of private pain.

The second critical point is that the subjective quality of nociceptive innervation, not the physical quality of such innervation, serves to subjectively punish trial-and-error responses that aggravate or perpetuate sensations of pain and to subjectively reward trial-and-error responses that successfully defy or reduce sensations of pain. Accordingly, if an organism's sensations suddenly include painful ones, and if the organism judges the painful sensations to be *intolerable*, then the judgment's physical aspects (paralleling its subjective aspects) can serve as a neural trigger for generating trial-and-error responses to the painful sensations. Ultimately, if the organism generates a pain-reducing or pain-defying response, and if the organism subjectively reevaluates its pain as less intense or more tolerable, then the reevaluation's physical aspects can serve as a neural signal for committing to the particular response. The variability inherent in this process, wherein different individuals tolerate different levels of any pain that they are not innately equipped to escape, promotes survival of the species.

On this account, during the evolution of early animals with primitive nervous systems, *intolerable sensations of pain* reinforced the trial-and-error neural development of pain-escaping reflexes, which are preserved in mammals' spinal reflexes to escape pain and as such are responsible for the pain-escaping behaviors of decerebrated mammals (Clarke, Wych, & Harris, 2001; Schouenborg, Holmberg, & Weng, 1992; Sherrington, 1911). And during the evolution of early mammals with a neocortex, *tolerable pain* that interfered with competing demands fostered the neural development of corticofugal pathways for inhibiting the spine's pain-escaping reflexes (Hutchison, Harfa, & Dostrovsky, 1996; Pavlov, 1927).

As we continue, it is important to keep in mind that when painful sensations evolved into visual sensations, auditory sensations, and other sensations, the reinforcement quality of pain was not passed on. Neither brightness per se nor yellowness per se is subjectively reinforcing. So when students of consciousness ask whether conscious sensations have any causal effects on thought or behavior, we can give an affirmative reply with regard to painful sensation, but we cannot give an affirmative reply regarding any sensation that has evolved from pain.

PAIN AS THE SUBJECTIVE ASPECT OF FREE NERVE ENDINGS OR NOCICEPTORS

The preceding argument for the causal efficacy of painful sensations is predicated on the assumption that pain is the subjective quality of nociceptors—primitive sensory receptors that are essentially free nerve endings—and is not the subjective quality of more recently evolved cortical neurons. For a long time, research on human pain failed to confirm that sensations of pain correspond to the discharges of nociceptors, and pain researchers concluded that pain resulted from a CNS computation based not only on nociceptive input but also on emotional and cognitive input. But three decades ago, Robinson, Torebjörk, and LaMotte (1983) and Torebjörk, LaMotte, and Robinson (1984) examined microneurographical recordings of the electrical discharge from single nociceptors in humans, and they confirmed that the absolute threshold and the subjective magnitude of painful sensation correspond, respectively, to the onset and the frequency of nociceptor discharge during noxious heat stimulation. And in more recent research with human participants, Schmidt, Schmelz, Torebjörk, and Handwerker (2000) confirmed that the threshold and magnitude of pain correspond also to the onset and the frequency of nociceptor discharge during noxious pressure stimulation. Notably, most nociceptors are embedded in the skin. However, recent research indicates that nociceptors are also embedded in the intestines, the heart, and the testes (Feinle, 1998; Hisata, Zeredo, Eishi, & Toda, 2006; Yoshioka, Tanahashi, & Uchida, 2010). In addition, muscle-innervating nerve terminals that are unmyelinated tend to serve as nociceptors during painful stretching or contracting of a muscle, and joint-innervating nerve terminals that are exposed tend to serve as nociceptors during painful movement outside the normal range (Millan, 1999). And in studies with implications for the evolution of nociceptors, pain researcher Marshall Devor (2006) found that midnerve damage causes axons to respond the way free nerve endings respond to noxious stimulation, and pain researcher Peter Reeh applied noxious heat to an exposed axon in his superficial radial nerve and experienced a sensation of burning pain (Devor, 2009; Hoffmann, Sauer, Horch, Reeh, & Hoffmann, 2009).

Cases of phantom pain in the missing limb of a human amputee, when taken simply at face value, are often interpreted as showing that painful sensation is a subjective CNS quality rather than a subjective aspect of the nociceptor. Moving beyond this simplistic interpretation, however, psychophysiological studies of amputees demonstrate that phantom sensations are paralleled by neural activity in the stump's sensory transmitters, as well as by neural activity in the CNS's body schema, wherein the missing limb is represented and is associated with the stump's sensations. In young amputees whose CNS representation of the missing limb has not developed, in older amputees whose CNS representation of the missing limb has atrophied, and in cortically damaged amputees whose schematic representation of the missing limb has been destroyed, phantom sensations are not experienced (Cronholm, 1951; Katz, 1993, 2000; Ramachandran & Hirstein, 1998). Neural activity in the stump's sensory transmitters and parallel "phantom sensations" can be elicited by pricking the stump, can be extinguished by anesthetizing the stump, and can be measured concurrently (Cronholm, 1951; Katz, 1992, 1993; Ramachandran & Hirstein, 1998). Thus, the psychophysiological data concerning phantom sensation are consistent with this chapter's thesis that painful sensations and all other sensations are the subjective aspects of sensory transmitters, along with its corollary that all subjective aspects conveying locative information are the sensationless aspects of CNS schemata and as such are tacitly apprehended in relation to particular sensations.

THE EVOLUTION OF PRESSURE, HEAT, AND CHEMICAL NOCICEPTORS IN PRIMITIVE NERVOUS SYSTEMS

Over 650 million years ago, the animal phylum Porifera (sponges) emerged with no nervous system and, hence, no free nerve endings with a subjectively painful quality that happened to occur during their innervation and happiness to promote survival.subjectively painful quality that happens to occur during their innervation and happens to promote survival. Eventually, at least 500 million years ago, four animal phyla with primitive nervous systems evolved: the phylum Cnidaria (corals, anemones, jellyfish), the phylum Platyhelminthes (tapeworms, flukes, flatworms), the phylum Annelida (earthworms, ragworms, leeches), and the phylum Nematoda (roundworms) (see Wang, Kumar, & Hedges, 1999). Then, over 350 million years ago, three neurally more advanced phyla evolved: the phylum Mollusca (octopus, squid, slugs, snails), the phylum Anthropoda (crustaceans, arachnids, insects), and the fish family Salmonidae (salmon, chars, whitefish, graylings, trout).

In sea anemones and marine flatworms, scientists have been able to elicit nociceptive responses to noxious pressure stimuli but have been unable to differentiate nociceptive neurons (Smith & Lewin, 2009); in leeches, roundworms, snails, fruit flies, and trout, scientists have identified pressure nociceptors (de Bono & Maricq, 2005; Nicholls & Baylor, 1968; Pastor, Soria, & Belmonte, 1996; Sneddon, Braithwaite, & Gentle, 2003; Walters, 2009; Zhong, 2012). In leeches, snails, fruit flies, and trout, scientists have identified heat nociceptors (Kalil-Gaspar, Marcuzzo, Rigon, Molina, & Achaval, 2007; Pastor et al., 1996; Sneddon et al., 2003; Zhong, 2012). And in leeches, roundworms, snails, fruit flies, and trout, researchers have identified chemical nociceptors (de Bono & Maricq, 2005; Kalil-Gaspar et al., 2007; Kang et al., 2010; Pastor et al., 1996; Sneddon et al., 2003). Inasmuch as the pressure nociceptor and the heat nociceptor and the chemical nociceptor promote survival, it seems reasonable to assume that at least one of these three categories of free nerve endings will ultimately be identified in all animals with nervous systems including those with primitive nervous systems that can neither see nor hear.

Before turning our attention to the central thesis of this chapter—that chemical, pressure, and heat nociceptors evolved into taste receptors, touch receptors, and temperature receptors, respectively—let us note that pain plays a role not only in the evolution of sensations but also in the evolution of sentiments or emotions. Indeed, in his classic book, *The Expression of the Emotions in Man and Animals*, Charles Darwin (1872/2009) maintained that "Pain, if severe, soon induces extreme depression" (p. 85). The role of pain in negative emotions is discussed in Appendix B of this book.

CHEMICAL NOCICEPTORS AS SUBSTRUCTURES FROM WHICH TASTE AND SMELL RECEPTORS EVOLVED

In research on gustatory nociception in Drosophila (commonly known as fruit flies), Al-Anzi, Tracey, and Benzer (2006) uncovered evidence indicating that mutations in three specific alleles serve to transform a chemical nociceptor into a gustatory receptor or taste receptor. In the first phase of this research, some normal fruit flies and some fruit flies mutant for the alleles $pain^{1}$, $pain^{2}$, and $pain^{GAL4}$ were food deprived, then were exposed to a food tray containing both a harmless sugary liquid and a sugary liquid laced with the insecticide isothiocyanate. Whereas the normal fruit flies consumed the harmless sugary liquid and avoided the sugary insecticide, the mutant flies consumed both the harmless sugary liquid and the sugary insecticide. In the second phase, through differential fluorescent labeling of neurons with the $pain^{GAL4}$ mutation and neurons with various gustatory receptors, the researchers were able to confirm that some of the neurons expressing the $pain^{GAL4}$ mutation also expressed the gustatory neuron reporter Gr66a-GFP. Thus, in fruit flies that were products of an experimentally induced mutation, gustatory receptors manifesting bitterness without pain "evolved" from chemical nociceptors manifesting painful bitterness.

In five Drosophila species sharing a common ancestor around 12 million years ago, gustatory receptors for specific tastes have evolved along the lines of species-specific mutations (McBride & Arguello, 2007). In humans, sweet-taste receptors are encoded by TAS1R2 and TAS1R3 genes, and individual differences in sweet reception are encoded by mutant alleles on these two genes (Kim, Wooding, Riaz, Jorde, & Drayna, 2006); umami taste receptors are encoded by TAS1R1 and TAS1R3 genes, and individual differences in umami reception are encoded by mutant alleles on these genes (Chen et al., 2009; Raliou et al., 2009); bitter taste receptors are encoded by TAS2R genes, and individual differences in bitter reception are encoded by mutant alleles thereon (Kim, Wooding, Ricci, Jorde, & Drayna, 2005; Li, Pakstis, Kidd, & Kidd, 2011); sour taste receptors are encoded by ASIC and PKD genes, and individual differences in sour reception are encoded by mutant alleles on these genes (Huque et al., 2009).

Some ancient species with the most primitive nervous systems—various species of coral, in particular—appear to have gustatory receptors for a few basic tastes and not to have olfactory receptors for any of the many differentiable odors (Kass-Simon & Hufnagel, 1992; Reimer, 1971; Satterlie & Case, 1978). Other early species with more evolved, but still primitive, nervous systems—various species of snail, for example—exhibit both gustatory receptors and olfactory receptors (Chase & Tolloczko, 1993; Kamardin, Shalanki, Rozha, &

Nozdrachev, 2001; Nakamura et al., 1999; M. Voss, 2000). This leads us to infer that olfactory chemoreceptors probably evolved as mutant forms of gustatory chemoreceptors. Of course, if species with olfactory chemoreceptors but no gustatory chemoreceptors can be documented, then we should infer instead that olfactory receptors probably evolved independently of gustatory receptors as mutant forms of chemical nociceptors.

PRESSURE NOCICEPTORS AS SUBSTRUCTURES FROM WHICH TOUCH AND SOUND RECEPTORS EVOLVED

In Tracey, Wilson, Laurent, and Benzer's (2003) research on the genetics of nociception in *Drosophila* larvae, nociceptors with a high threshold for innervation by mechanical pressure were transformed by a $pain^{1}$-allele mutation into low-threshold mechanoreceptors or touch receptors. In the course of evolution, moreover, the free nerve endings of pressure nociceptors have mutated into four different end organs—Pacinian corpuscles, Meissner's corpuscles, Merkel's disks, and Ruffini endings—in the tactile mechanoreceptors or touch receptors that give rise to sensations of pressure, vibration, and texture (Bolanowski, Gescheider, Verrillo, & Checkosky, 1988; McGlone & Reilly, 2010). Pacinian corpuscles are innervated by tactile contact with physical vibrations in the 40–500 Hz range and, in that they respond primarily to initial and final contact, are fast-adapting mechanoreceptors. Meisser's corpuscles are innervated by tactile contact with physical vibrations in the 2–40 Hz range and also are fast-adapting receptors. Merkel's disks are innervated by tactile contact with physical pressures in the 0.4–2.0 Hz range and, in that they respond continuously during stimulation, are slowly adapting mechanoreceptors. Ruffini endings are innervated by tactile contact with physical vibrations in the 100–500 Hz range and also are slowly adapting receptors.

Additional research suggests that the pressure nociceptor's free nerve endings, in addition to evolving into these four sensory transmitters for cutaneous touch, have mutated into free nerve endings that are discriminably different from nociceptors (Schmelz, 2010) and are apparently associated with subjective qualities like itch, tickle, and sexual pleasure (Cooper, 1972; Nafe, 1927; Schmelz, Schmidt, Bickel, Handwerker, & Torebjörk, 1997). With regard to male sexual pleasure, Cooper (1972) discovered that male snails have contact-innervated free nerve endings on their glans penis; and with regard to female sexual pleasure, Sakai, Kasuya, Kitamoto and Aigaki (2009) discovered that female fruit flies with $pain^{1}$, $pain^{2}$, and $pain^{GAL4}$ mutations copulate significantly earlier than normal female fruit flies. We can safely infer that the reproduction-promoting pleasure innervated by tactile contact with free nerve endings on the genitals evolved after, if not from, the nociceptor's free nerve endings, given that the corals, anemones, and jellyfish belonging to the oldest surviving phylum of animals exhibit nociception but do not exhibit either courtship or copulation.[6]

In accordance with this chapter's hypothesis that auditory mechanoreceptors evolved from tactile mechanoreceptors, Eberl, Hardy, and Kernan's (2000) research on fruit flies has confirmed that mutations in some genes diminish sensitivity both to sound and to touch. More primitive animals such as flatworms, roundworms, and leeches cannot detect sound pressure (Budelmann, 1992) but can detect tactile pressure (Blackshaw, Nicholls, & Parnas, 1982; Watson & Rohde, 1994; Wright, 1977). And unlike the fruit fly, many insect species cannot detect sound pressure (Yager, 1999), although all insect species can detect tactile pressure (Keil, 1997). Presumably, as tactile mechanoreceptors mutated into auditory mechanoreceptors capable of detecting airborne and waterborne waves of sound pressure, the subjective "touch qualities" of tactile pressure receptors mutated into the subjective "sound qualities" of auditory pressure receptors. And by implication, given that fundamental physical aspects of sound-pressure reception are conserved in the tympanate ears of insects and reptiles and mammals (Manley, 2000; Yager, 1999), the fundamental subjective aspects of auditory sensation should be conserved as well.

HEAT NOCICEPTORS AS SUBSTRUCTURES FROM WHICH TEMPERATURE AND LIGHT RECEPTORS EVOLVED

In studying heat nociception in adult fruit flies, Xu et al. (2006) found that normal fruit flies walk away from mildly aversive warmth and fly away from more noxious heat, whereas fruit flies with *pain[1]* mutations walk away from both—a finding that suggests that the mutants' heat nociceptors were transformed into temperature receptors. And in studying temperature sensing in roundworms, fruit flies, and mice, David McKemy (2007) came to the conclusion that the molecular mediators of temperature sensation in worms and flies' nervous systems are conserved in mammals' nervous systems.

Evidence to date suggests that the first neural receptor capable of sensing light was the jellyfish's ocellus (Parker, 2003; Schwab, 2012). Like the light-stimulated organs that Parker (2003) and Schwab (2012) describe in plants and in one-celled animals, the light-stimulated ocelli in jellyfish are capable of influencing behavior in the absence of a brain (Nordström, Wallén, Seymour, and Nilsson, 2003).[7] Notwithstanding the ocellus's brainless functioning, the *PaxB* gene encoding its physical aspects has apparently mutated into the *Pax6* gene encoding physical aspects of the primitive eyespots of flatworms (Gehring, 1996; Kozmik, 2008), as well as physical aspects of the highly evolved eyes of human beings and various birds (Bandah et al., 2007; Schwab, 2012). Planarian eyespots contain photoreceptive cells with only one photopigment, rhodopsin (Davidson et al., 2011), whereas human and avian eyes contain brightness-discriminating *rod cells* with rhodopsin as well as three to four types of color-discriminating *cone cells* with opsin-based photopigments.[8]

Interestingly, the flatworm does not see any visual images of objects that reflect light onto its eyespot, because it has not evolved a lens or any other means of focusing light (Parker, 2003; Smales & Blankespoor, 1978). So what is the function of the flatworm's eyespot? In studies by Davidson et al. (2011) and Pescetto and Dettore (1981), flatworms' eyespots acted like light-triggered nociceptors and evoked avoidance behaviors in response to intense light, presumably because such intense "airborne heat" triggered subjectively painful qualities in the eyespots.

Thus, it seems likely that warm-blooded animals' retinal cells, which are physically responsive to various intensities and wavelengths of light, evolved from light nociceptors or "airborne heat" nociceptors similar to flatworms' unseeing eyespots. Presumably, eyespots diverged not only into rod and cone cells but also into simple and compound eyes. And eventually, simple eyes with both rods and cones diverged into fish eyes with three to seven cone types, avian eyes with four cone types, sea-mammal eyes with one cone type, and human eyes with three cone types (Bowmaker, 2008; Hunt, Carvalho, Cowing, & Davies, 2009; Larhammar, Nordström, & Larsson, 2009). As we move forward and consider the human visual system in more detail, it is important to remember that only the physical aspects of this system can have adaptive value and that the subjective aspects of this system, unlike the subjective aspects of nociceptors, do not have such value. For instance, the physical responsiveness of cone cells to a plant reflecting 400 nm lightwaves can signal the central nervous system (CNS) not to eat the potentially poisonous plant. However, the subjective aspect of a purplish plant does not have the intrinsically reinforcing effect that the subject aspect of painful food poisoning has. Accordingly, the conscious sensation of purple is epiphenomenal, even though the painful sensation paralleling the type of nociceptor that evolved into purple-responsive cone cells is not an epiphenomenon.

Let us begin, then, with the three types of cone cells in the normal human eye's retina. The short-wavelength (S) cone cells are responsive within a mini-spectrum that peaks at stimulating lightwaves of 435 nm and at paralleling sensations of blue-violet; medium-wavelength (M) cone cells are responsive within a different mini-spectrum that peaks at stimulating lightwaves of 530 nm and at paralleling sensations of greenness; and long-wavelength (L) cone cells are responsive within a third mini-spectrum that peaks at stimulating lightwaves of 560 nm and at paralleling sensations of yellow-green, as Figure 2 indicates.

The S cone cell's photopigment proteins differ from the M cone cell's photopigment proteins, and both the S cone cell's and M cone cell's photopigment proteins differ from the L cone cell's photopigment proteins. Eugene Brooks (2011–2012) suggests "that the protein expressed by the gene in [cone cells with peak responsiveness to 435 nm lightwaves] fills the role of the somatic basis for

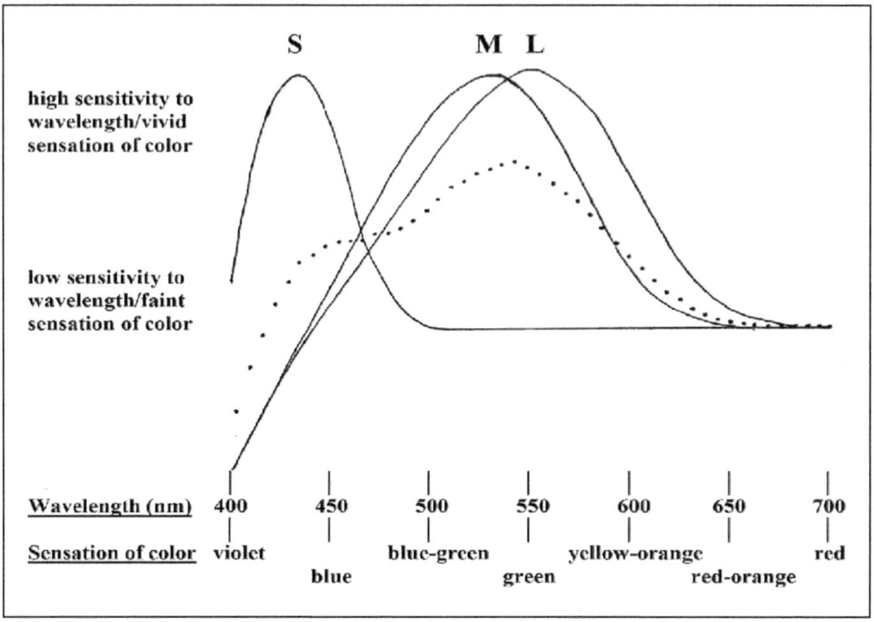

Figure 2. The short-wavelength (S) cone cell's mini-spectrum ranging from low-level 400 nm sensitivity paralleled by faint violet sensation, to 435 nm peak sensitivity paralleled by vivid blue-violet sensation, to low-level 475 nm sensitivity paralleled by faint blue sensation; the medium-wavelength (M) cone cell's mini-spectrum ranging from low-level 435 nm sensitivity paralleled by faint blue-violet sensation, to 530 nm peak sensitivity paralleled by vivid green sensation, to low-level 625 nm sensitivity paralleled by faint red-orange sensation; and the long-wavelength (L) cone cell's mini-spectrum ranging from low-level 450 nm sensitivity paralleled by faint blue sensation, to 560 nm peak sensitivity paralleled by vivid yellow-green sensation, to low-level 700 nm sensitivity paralleled by faint red sensation. The dotted curve plots the mean photopic sensitivity (S + M + L/3) at each wavelength of light.

a quality [where the] quality expressed is the perception of light in the blue range" (p. 218) and overall suggests "that *certain proteins have the unexpected and amazing characteristics of being sensations, that is, the characteristics of being* [*subjective*] *qualities*" (p. 230). Brooks' suggestions not only point to the particular physical aspects that apparently parallel particular sensations of color, but also point to some broader implications regarding the physical and subjective aspects of cone-cell functioning.

One of these implications is that each type of cone cell cannot have just one subjective aspect manifested as one sensation of color but must have a subjective mini-spectrum of colorful sensations—in accord with Hofer, Singer, and Williams' (2005) finding that human "photoreceptors within the same [L, M, or S] class can elicit more than one color sensation . . . [indeed] a wide variety of color sensation" in response to single-cone stimulation by light-waves associated with medium-bandwidth color (p. 444). Thus as Figure 2 illustrates, the various photopigment proteins stimulated in S cones should have subjective aspects ranging from faint violet sensations for 400 nm stimuli in the left tail of sensitivity, to vivid blue-violet sensations for 435 nm stimuli at peak sensitivity, to faint blue sensations for 475 nm stimuli in the right tail of sensitivity. In contrast, the various photopigment proteins stimulated in M cones should have subjective aspects ranging from faint blue-violet sensations for 435 nm stimuli in the left tail of sensitivity, to vivid green sensations for 530 nm stimuli at peak sensitivity, to faint red-orange sensations for 625 nm stimuli in the right tail of sensitivity. In addition, the various photopigment proteins stimulated in L cones should have subjective aspects ranging from faint blue sensations for 450 nm stimuli in the left tail of sensitivity, to vivid yellow-green sensations for 560 nm stimuli at peak sensitivity, to faint red sensations for 700 nm stimuli in the right tail of sensitivity. And when mean photopic sensitivity (S + M + L/3) is plotted for each wavelength of visible light, as has been plotted in Figure 2's dotted curve, the result matches rather well J. J. Voss' (1978) photopic sensitivity function—a function indicating that the normal human eye is most sensitive to 550 nm green-yellow and least sensitive to 400 nm purple and 700 nm red.

Notably, because the firing rate of cones is the only neural signal they can transmit regarding their subjectively colorful quality (i.e., because a slower "M cone" firing rate could be subjectively paralleled by a faint blue retinal quality or by a faint orange retinal quality), the brain requires signals from adjacent S, M, and L cones in order to make a sensationless inference about the particular color that parallels all three cones, at cone-specific degrees of saturation. The neural signals generated by S, M, and L cones are transmitted to retinal ganglion cells and the lateral geniculate nucleus for sensationless encoding into red/green and yellow/blue polarities, which are subsequently encoded by the primary visual cortex into hue-specific neural signals and are finally encoded by visual area 4 (V4) of the striate cortex into signals specifying color constancies (Komatsu, 1998). Given that local retinal color implicates different color constancies in different global contexts (as both the introspectionists and the Gestalt psychologists have made clear), these final signals in area V4 allow us to make sensationless inferences about context-influenced color constancies at the same time that the retina's subjectively colorful aspects allow us locally to introspect context-free sensations of color.[9]

The above account stands in contrast to arguments for "the cortical construction of color" in the brain's "color center" (Heywood & Kentridge, 2003, p. 496). Semir Zeki (2001) argues that, in humans, this "color center is located in the fusiform gyrus and consists of two subdivisions, V4 and V4α" (p. 63), and Lawrence Weiskrantz (2002) argues that, in this color center, a "mixture generated by the inputs from two eyes merging together upstream, red from one eye and green from the other is yellow—so-called 'cortical yellow'" (p. 577). However, Hurvich and Jameson (1951) and Kunzendorf (2007b, 2009) have shown that the binocular perception of red light in one eye and green light in the other yields yellow sensations only when wide-bandwidth red light containing some yellow light and wide-bandwidth green light containing some yellow light are stereoscopically presented, not when narrow-bandwidth red light containing no yellow light and narrow-bandwidth green light containing no yellow light are stereoscopically presented. Moreover, Kunzendorf (2014) has rapidly rotated wide-bandwidth red and green light, as well as narrow-bandwidth red and green light in order to better understand the monocular mixture of yellow, which has been studied since the 19th century by rapidly spinning either a toy top or a flat disc that is half red and half green (Ihara & Kido, 1935; Maxwell, 1855; Scripture, 1895). For a long time, only wide-bandwidth red and green stimuli were amenable to spinning, as narrow-bandwidth red and green had to be generated through non-rotatable prisms. But recently, using modern light filters with wide and narrow bandwidths, Kunzendorf (2014) has found that sensations of yellow are visible only when a wide-bandwidth red light and a wide-bandwidth green light are rapidly rotated. When a narrow-bandwidth red light and a narrow-bandwidth green light are rapidly rotated, only color sensations of interspersed red and green are visible, along with some white sensations that are attributable to rod-cell responsiveness to red light and green light (Baylor, Lamb, & Yau, 1979; Palacios & Goldsmith, 1993). This narrow-bandwidth finding disconfirms the constructivist position that yellow sensations are mixed in the cortex upon its receipt of retinofugal signals triggered by S, M, and L cone cells' sensationless responses to rapidly alternating red and green lights of any bandwidth. For wide-bandwidth "mixtures" of yellow, all that needs to be posited by way of noncortical explanation is that the retinal activation of both yellow and red sensations in L cones, alternating with the retinal activation of both the subjectively yellow aspects and the subjectively green aspects of M cones, yields sensations of yellow twice as often as sensations of either green or red.[10] And most important to our understanding of the physical and phenomenal functioning of the human cortex, what emerge in cortical area V4 are sensationless inferences about color constancy—inferences that are subjectively experienced in relation to the colorful subjective aspects of stimulated cone cells in the retina. Accordingly, area V4's sensationless inferences regarding color constancy dispose us to behave as if an apple composed of bright red sensations in the context of sunlight and the same apple composed of dark red sensations in the context of shade are one and the same apple with inferred redness constancy.

SENSATIONLESS CORTICAL INFERENCES REGARDING CONSCIOUS SENSATIONS

The cortical calculation of color constancy from colorful sensations and their context can be readily appreciated if one rests both of one's index fingers on a uniformly brightly colored surface and then casts one's own shadow all over and all around the left index finger. By introspectively focusing on the colorful sensations composing each finger, one can subjectively appreciate the left finger's qualitatively darker sensations of color. One's mind nevertheless, in addition to containing the two fingers' qualitatively different sensations of color, contains the sensationless cortical inference that the two fingers' colors are constant, based on V4 computations equating the left finger's S-cone, M-cone, and L-cone firing frequencies in a shadowy context and the right finger's quantitatively different firing frequencies in a shadowless context.

In persons who are "color blind" for red and green, either mutated L cones exhibit peak responsiveness to 545 nm green-yellow instead of 560 nm yellow-green, or mutated M cones exhibit peak responsiveness to 545 nm green-yellow instead of 530 nm green (Jordan, Deeb, Boston, & Mollon, 2010). Thus, in the color-blind person's cortex, any and all attempts inferentially to discriminate red and green are based on L-cone signals and M-cone signals with abnormally close overlap and are likely to fail. But as Justin Broackes (2010) documents in his chapter "What Do the Color-Blind See?", the color--blind person's retina still produces sensations that are experienced as red and green, even though they are not cortically discriminable. Indeed, a color-blind friend of mine tells me that when he looks for the numbers in Shinobu Ishihara's (1962) color-blindness test, he can focus on one of the colored dots composing a number and can experience its redness or greenness, but literally cannot "connect the dots" and cannot identify the red-and-green-dotted number. As noted in Broackes' chapter, "Discriminating red and green is one thing; actually seeing—or having sensations of—red and green is another" (p. 295).

Color constancy is just one among many constancies that the cortex computes in relation to visually perceived sensations. Size constancy is another, which one can appreciate by holding up both index fingers in front of one's eyes—the left finger 10 inches away from one's left eye, and the right finger 20 inches away from one's right eye. By introspectively focusing on the vertical size of the sensations composing each finger, one can phenomenally experience the vertical size of left-finger sensations as twice that of right-finger sensations. But in addition to containing left- and right-finger sensations of different phenomenal size, one's mind contains the sensationless inference that the two finger's vertical sizes in reality are constant, based on cortical calculations equating the left finger's retinal size from a depth of 10 inches and the right finger's retinal size from a depth of 20 inches. Depth-related inferences tend to be computationally intertwined with size-related inferences in adult human beings, to the extent that their visual cortexes have developed the computational rules of 2-point and 3-point perspective (Kunzendorf & Buker, 2008–2009; Kunzendorf et al., 2012–2013). In children, on the other hand, depth-related inferences tend not to be in sync with size-related inferences, inasmuch as children's inferences regarding depth are based on partial visual occlusion rather than linear perspective (Granrud, 2009; Mandes, 1985; Olson, 1975; Shukla & Sinha, 1974).

In addition to computing such constancies, the cortex usually computes the bodily location or spatial location from which a sensation is tacitly inferred to arise. Earlier in this chapter, our consideration of phantom sensations showed us how the sensations paralleling activated receptors in amputees' stumps can be tacitly inferred to arise in missing limbs that are still cortically represented in the amputees' body schemas. Cortical lesions inducing allochiria —the mislocation of a painful sensation or a tactile sensation on the opposite side of the body (Bender, Shapiro, & Teuber, 1949; Jones, 1908; Venneri, Pentore, Cobelli, Nichelli, & Shanks, 2012)—further illustrate that the *sensory quality* of a nociceptor or a mechanoreceptor is subjectively separate from its tacitly associated *locative aspect*, the cortical underpinnings of which inform motoric dispositions in relation to the sensory quality.

With regard to sensationless aspects of spatial location, their phenomenal separability from visual sensations is best illustrated by Skavensky, Haddad, and Steinman's (1972) research findings. Both of the human subjects in their research had a scleral contact lens suctioned onto one eye and looked through that eye into a darkened laboratory with a fixation point visible straight ahead, while weights connected to a stalk on the contact lens exerted a leftward pull on the eye. When asked to position an out-of-view object directly underneath the visible fixation point (while using their eye muscles to counter the leftward pull and to keep their eye focused on the fixation point), subjects positioned the object at a cortically calculated "straight ahead" spatial location to the right of the fixation point that was actually straight ahead. When the leftward force pulling on their eye was maximized, the subjects kept their eye focused straight ahead on the fixation point, but cortically calculated "straight ahead" to be 15°–20° to the right of the fixation point (e.g., far beyond the 6° rightward edge of normal reading material). Thus, their cortex's calculation of the spatial location of the fixation point took into account the muscular feedback from their pulled eye and yielded sensationless locative knowledge in relation to (but separable from) the retinal sensation stimulated by the fixation point.

Like the sensationless aspects of color constancy, size constancy, depth, bodily location, spatial location, and other *perceptual inferences*, the sensationless aspects of many *conceptual inferences* are experienced in relation to sensations, but less directly so, given that conceptual inferences tend to be mediated by perceptual inferences. For example, the concept of density—weight per unit volume—is mediated by perceptual rules for inferring weight constancy from muscular sensations of pressure and by perceptual rules for inferring volume constancy from visual sensations' height, width, and depth constancies (Brainerd, 1971; Luu, Day, Cole, & Fitzpatrick, 2011; Piaget & Inhelder, 1947, 1971). Thus, developmentally, children cannot conceptually understand why a 2-pound bag of sand has greater density than a 5-pound wooden log until after they can parse their sensations into perceptual constancies of weight and volume. Of course, fully developed adults can understand why a 200-pound bag of sand has greater density than a 500-pound wooden log, even though they cannot directly sense the weight of either. But in such adults, the sensationless concept of density can be experienced *either* in relation to sensations that are directly perceived *or* in relation to sensations that, based on extrapolations from cortical rules, are hypothetically possible. And as Oswald Külpe (1893/1895, p. 206), Ulric Neisser (1976), Jean Piaget (1972), and Xenon Pylyshyn (1973, 1981, 2003) have duly noted, adults can anticipate the sensory possibilities implied by any rule, perceptual or conceptual, without generating mentally imaged sensations.[11]

Sometimes, the tacitly known meaning of density is experienced symbolically—when one reads a map coding low, median, and high population densities as yellow, orange, and red, for example, or when one reads a scattergraph plotting cities according to their population density on the y-axis and their distance from a body of fresh water on the x-axis. As a graph of the latter sort is read, the sensationless concept of density, on one hand, is experienced in relation to perceptual sensations of the graph and, on the other hand, is understood in relation to possible sensations of "people per city block" as they co-vary with possible sensations of "distance from fresh water."

In relation to the *mentally imaged* sensation (the focus of Chapter 3), the cortex can calculate that the neural origin of such a sensation is central, not peripheral; and subjectively paralleling this cortical calculation of origin is the tacit inference that *one is imaging the sensation* (Kunzendorf, 1985–1986a, 1992–1993; Kunzendorf, Moran, & Gray, 1995–1996). Self-consciousness—the illusion of one's self as a "subject of consciousness" who is *having* a sensation (the focus of Chapter 4)—is the generic relational experience arising either from the tacit knowledge that *one is perceiving a sensation* or from the tacit knowledge that *one is imaging a sensation* (Kunzendorf, 1987–1988; 2000). And because self-consciousness is a sensationless cortical phenomenon in relation to (but separate from) all introspected sensations, David Hume (1739/1896) was able to make his famous introspection-based assertion:

> For my part, when I enter most intimately into what I call *myself,* I always stumble on some particular [sensation] or other, of heat or cold, light or shade, love or hatred, pain or pleasure. I never can catch *myself* at any time without a [sensation], and never can observe anything but the [sensation]. (Bk. I, Pt. IV, Sec. VI, p. 134)

Further evidence that the subjective aspects of all cortical calculations are sensationless,[12] and are experienced only *in relation to* sensations paralleling the activation of sensory transmitters, comes from the scientific literature on sensations in decorticate mammals (Bard & Rioch, 1937; Denton, McKinley, Farrell, & Egan, 2009; Merker, 2007; Shewmon, Holmes, & Byrne, 1999). In Bard and Rioch's (1937) study of a cat whose cerebral cortex was surgically removed in two stages, the cat sniffed when nearby foods stimulated its olfactory receptors with their parallel sensations of smell, and it oriented its head when noises stimulated its cochlear receptors with their parallel sensations of sound. In

Shewmon et al.'s (1999) study of four human children whose hydraencephaly made them congenitally decorticate, all four children smiled or giggled when their favorite music stimulated sensations of sound in their cochleae. And in one decorticate child, the sight of bright light evoked both retinal potentials and blinking reflexes (even though it evoked no posterior waveforms), and the visual sensation of a toy evoked smiling and giggling. Such studies are consistent with this chapter's two theses: that sensations are the subjective qualities of sensory receptors, and that calculations in the subcortex—and in whatever cortex has developed—are subjectively experienced as sensationless inferences in relation to the sensations from which they are computed. By implication, after retinal projections are surgically rerouted into primary auditory cortex, as in research by Roe, Pallas, Hahm, and Sur (1990), the retina's subjective aspects are still visual sensations, but going forward, the spatial mapping of those visual sensations is in the sensationless auditory cortex.

EPILOGUE: LEAPFROGGING 20TH CENTURY BIASES

As we have seen, both 19th century theorizing and 21st century evidence is consistent with this chapter's main thesis: that free nerve endings, with subjectively painful qualities yielding a survival advantage, evolved into complex receptors like retinae and cochlea, with subjective qualities of visual and auditory sensation having no causal efficacy. However, the theoretical biases inherent in early 20th century behavioral science, later 20th century cognitive science, and early 21st century neuroscience run counter to any such thesis.

During the first half of the 20th century, behavioral scientists like Max Meyer (1922) abandoned introspective study of oneself for third-person study of "the other one." During the second half of the 20th century, the computer metaphor for mind "brought psychologists out of the rat maze, into the metaphoric world of short-term memory stores, long-term memory searches, script-based inferences, and so on . . . [but did] not bring psychologists any closer to understanding consciousness" (Kunzendorf, 1990–1991, p. 106). And in the 21st century, neuroscientists like Chun Siong Soon and John-Dylan Haynes demonstrated that brain functions several seconds prior to a conscious decision determine the decision, and concluded that the brain is determinative and consciousness is epiphenomenal (Soon, Brass, Heinze, & Haynes, 2008; Soon, He, Bode, & Haynes, 2013).

Whereas behavioral science's starting point is the observation of external behavior (including one's own behavior in the case of radical behaviorism), cognitive science's starting point is the computer-metaphoric modeling of internal behavior or functioning; and neuroscience's starting point is the observation of internal behavior or functioning in the brain. But despite their different starting points, behavioral science, cognitive science, and neuroscience write off conscious sensations as epiphenomenal—because they have to do so. Behaviorism's founder John Watson (1913), in deeming mentally imaged sensations to be epiphenomenal, concedes that "if thought goes on in terms of centrally aroused sensations, as is maintained by the majority of both structural and functional psychologists, we should have to admit that there is a serious limitation on the side of method in behaviorism" (p. 421). Likewise, if any imaged sensation—or any perceived sensation such as pain—should ever have a causal effect on the human mind's internal functions or its overt behavior, then any scientific endeavor to reduce the human mind to a computer-like machine or a brain-like machine would be limited in method and doomed to fail. Accordingly, Susan Pockett (2004) and other neuroscientists who try to explain consciousness in this reductionist context suggest that consciousness is a brain-induced epiphenomenon with no causal effect on brain functioning. Similarly, Norman Dixon (1981), Euan Macphail (1998), and other cognitive scientists who try to explain consciousness in a reductionist context suggest that consciousness is an epiphenomenon that emerges after the unconscious machine-like processing of information is complete. Moreover, Macphail asserts that "there does not in fact seem to be any need for the experience of either pleasure or pain" and asks, "What *additional* function does pain serve that could not be served more simply by a direct link between signals from the classificatory system and the action systems?" (p. 14). But as implied earlier in this chapter, such assertive sophistry begs the question of how survival-promoting behaviors receive direction before a "direct link" develops or evolves; and in addition, it begs to be rebutted with a painful punch to the nose's nociceptors.

Thus, early 20th century behavioral science, latter 20th century cognitive science, and early 21st century neuroscience are biased against 19th century psychological science for theoretical reasons, not evidentiary reasons. No scientist in the 19th, 20th, or 21st century has discovered any mind-brain relationship that defies interpretation by 19th century psychological science or an updated understanding of it. Furthermore, the theoretically "objective" starting points of behavioral science, cognitive science, and neuroscience have neither discovery value nor interpretive value for serious students of the subjective aspects and corresponding physical aspects of our minds and nervous systems. In order to discover new data and reinterpret old data regarding such aspects, we must start with our conscious sensations, and we must generate hypotheses about both the physical objects stimulating particular sensations and the neural states possessing particular sensations as subjective qualities; then we must imaginally generate some of the sensations that are implied by our sensationsless hypotheses, must compare those imagined sensations against our actually perceived sensations, and must confirm or revise our hypotheses accordingly. Through this process, the current chapter's hypothesis regarding the evolution of conscious sensations has, indeed, led both to some newly discovered data concerning colorful subjective aspects of the human retina (e.g., Kunzendorf, 1984, 2014) and to many newly reinterpreted data pertaining to the evolution of conscious sensations from free nerve endings. As we turn our attention to conscious imagination in the next chapter, our evolutionary hypotheses will be guided by Külpe's (1893/1895) 19th century thesis that mental images are "centrally aroused sensations," localized in the sensory receptors and constructed from "imageless thoughts" in the cerebral cortex.

CHAPTER 3

The Evolution of Conscious Imagination

> As dogs, cats, horses, and probably all the higher animals, even birds have vivid dreams, and this is shewn by their movements and the sounds uttered, we must admit that they possess some power of imagination.
>
> —*The Descent of Man*, Charles Darwin (1879/2007, p. 122)

The current chapter is based on a three-pronged hypothesis: that mentally imaged sensations are the subjective qualities of corticofugally innervated neurons in the sensory transmitters, that corticofugally innervated sensations serve to test the adequacy of "imageless" perceptual rules under development in the central nervous system, and that the imaging of sensations and the development of rules occur only in warm-blooded animals with more highly evolved brains. The last of these assertions—that mental imaging occurs only in animals with highly evolved brains, as Darwin asserted in the quotation above—will be our starting point. Then, building on the thesis in Chapter 2 that sensations are the subjective qualities of sensory receptors, we will explore evidence suggesting that visually imaged sensations and auditorily imaged sensations are the subjective qualities of retinal neurons and cochlear neurons, respectively, both innervated by nerve signals traveling along corticofugal pathways from the central nervous system. Next, as we consider the function of individual and developmental differences in retinally imaged sensations, we will explore evidence indicating that vividly imaged sensations are constructed from imageless cortical rules in order to test the adequacy of newly hypothesized or newly refined rules. Finally, returning to the evolutionary implications of this chapter's tripartite hypothesis, we will consider scientific studies showing that the development of cortical rules—visuo-spatial rules for anticipating and parsing retinal sensations never visually perceived before, audio-temporal rules for anticipating and parsing cochlear sensations never auditorily perceived before—occurs only in warm-blooded animals.

THE EVOLUTION OF DREAMING AND IMAGING IN WARM-BLOODED ANIMALS

Research reveals that only warm-blooded animals—only mammals and birds—exhibit a period of sleep manifesting rapid eye movement or REM (Capellini, 2012; Hartmann, Bernstein, & Wilson, 1968; Low, Shank, Sejnowski, & Margoliash, 2008; Lyamin, Shpak, Nazarenko, & Mukhametov, 2002; McNamara, 2004; Nicol, Andersen, Phillips, & Berger, 2000; Rattenborg, 2006; Rattenborg, Amlaner, & Lima, 2000; J. M. Siegel, 2008; Siegel et al., 1999). And as classic studies by Aserinsky and Kleitman (1955) and Dement and Kleitman (1957) demonstrated, this period of REM sleep in humans is cyclical, normally recurring every 90–120 minutes throughout the night, and is associated with visual dreams that are usually remembered by the dreamer upon being awakened and queried shortly after REM sleep ends. The question of interest to us is whether such periods of REM sleep in other mammals and in birds are also indicative of dreaming.

Charles Vaughan's (1966) dissertation research employing a foot-shock-avoidance paradigm in sleeping monkeys provides the strongest evidence that other animals besides humans do dream during REM sleep. In Vaughan's study, rhesus monkeys were pretrained to press a bar rapidly in order to avoid electric shock—shock that started up whenever a pictorial image was projected into their darkened isolation chamber, but that turned off as long as their bar-pressing rate stayed at criterion for the duration of the picture. Following pretraining, the monkeys experienced total sensory isolation for 74–96 hours and, throughout their isolation, exhibited recurring periods of REM sleep. The National Institute of Mental Health's (1966) report on *Current Research on Sleep and Dreams* describes how the monkeys' pretraining interacted with their covert dreams during REM:

> During these rapid-eye-movement periods, the monkeys suddenly began pressing the bar at a frenetic pace, rapidly and regularly as in waking. Sometimes they also made facial grimaces, flared nostrils, breathed deeply, even barked as they pressed the bar. Presumably they were "seeing things" during these intervals of rapid eye movements and were avoiding the shock associated with images. After the isolation period was over, the monkeys were tested in the training situation to be sure they still responded reliably to the projected images. The investigators had seen only one instance of bar-pressing during waking, so they had little data about hallucinations, but the evidence that monkeys experience visual images in sleep was very strong. (p. 86)

It is important to note that both periodicity and eye movement are statistically associated not only with dreaming but also with wakeful imaging. Periodicity research by Wallace and Kokoszka (1995) indicates that the vividness of wakeful visual imagery waxes and wanes throughout the day, possibly in sync with the dream cycle and with the nervous system's ultradian rhythm. Eye-movement research by Laeng and Teodorescu (2002) indicates that the human eye's movements during wakeful imaging of a previously seen stimulus tend to "reenact" its movements during initial perception of the visual stimulus. Furthermore, research by Sima, Schultheis, and Barkowsky (2013) reveals that people exhibit spontaneous eye movements as they solve spatial problems, but only if they construct visual images while solving problems, not if their spatial thinking remains imageless. Likewise, we expect that warm-blooded animals not only tend to dream during REM sleep but also can image during wakefulness.

Indeed, scientists' observations of playful pretense in mammals provide evidence for wakeful imagination in nonhuman animals. Cathy Hayes (1951) and McCune and Agayoff (2002), for instance, reported on apes pretending that they were pulling imaginary pull-toys—pretense that surely involves tactile-muscular imagery and likely involves visual imagery as well. Lyn, Greenfield, and Savage-Rumbaugh (2006) reported on an ape named Panbanisha as she pretended to eat imaginary berries:

> Panbanisha "eats" directly off a picture of blueberries. She places her mouth onto the photograph, closes her lips while touching them to the picture, raises her head and makes mouth movements as if chewing. After a few repetitions of this behavior, Panbanisha then picks "blueberries" off of the picture with her fingers and "eats" them off her fingers—extending her mental representation of the pretend blueberries into visible space (i.e., away from the picture and her mouth). (p. 208)

Such pretend eating implicates tactile-muscular, gustatory, and visual imagery. In addition, Robert Mitchell (2013) reported on a "young dolphin [that], upon observing a person smoking at a window, swam to its mother and returned, spurting out milk from its mouth" (p. 479)—pretend smoking that entails visual imagination of a transformational nature.

At present, the evidence for waking imagery and dream imagery in warm-blooded animals is compelling, albeit not extensive. At the same time, no research whatsoever suggests that any cold-blooded animal can either image or dream. So let us turn our attention to evidence suggesting that the mentally imaged sensations under consideration in this chapter, like the conscious sensations considered in the last chapter, are subjective qualities of the sensory receptors.

THE CORTICOFUGAL INNERVATION OF MENTALLY IMAGED SENSATIONS

As noted in Chapter 1, Oswald Külpe (1893/1895) argued that, from imageless thoughts in the sensationless cortex, mental images are constructed in the sensory transmitters via corticofugally conducting nerves. Scientific evidence in support of Külpe's argument includes: (a) anatomical evidence that centrifugally conducting nerves terminate in the retina, the olfactory bulb, and the cochlea; (b) physiological evidence that micro-electrode stimulation of visual, olfactory, and auditory pathways in the central nervous system innervates the retina, the olfactory bulb, and the cochlea, respectively; and (c) psychophysiological evidence that visual imaging activates the retina, olfactory imaging the olfactory bulb, and auditory imaging the cochlea.

Anatomical Findings

Külpe (1893/1895) based his argument for centrifugally constructed images, in part, on Santiago Ramón y Cajal's (1888, 1889) anatomical evidence that the avian retina not only contains retinofugal nerves (which originate in the retina and ultimately innervate the pallium or avian cortex) but also contains retinopetal nerves (which terminate in the retina and presumably innervate it centrifugally or cortiofugally). Centrifugal nerve fibers terminating in the olfactory bulb were discovered around the same time in Yervante Manouélian's (1898) study of the feline and rodent olfactory systems, and centrifugal nerves terminating in the cochlea were discovered later in Grant Rasmussen's (1942, 1953) studies of the feline auditory system. Extending each of the above findings to the other class of warm-blooded animals, Alexander Dogiel (1895) found centrifugal nerves terminating in the dog retina; Reiner and Karten (1985) found centrifugal nerves terminating in the waterfowl olfactory bulb; and Robert Boord (1961) found centrifugal nerves terminating in the pigeon cochlea.

Throughout the second half of the 20th century, anatomical studies by Honrubia and Elliott (1968), Michiro Matsuyama (1967), Sacks and Lindenberg (1969), Ventura and Mathieu (1959, 1960), and Jurgen Reimer Wolter (1965a, 1965b, 1979, 1991) confirmed the existence of centrifugal nerves terminating in the human retina; research by Briñón et al. (1998) confirmed the existence of centrifugal nerves terminating in the human olfactory bulb; and studies by Richard Gacek (1961), Ishii, Murakami, and Balogh (1967), Nomura and Schuknecht (1965), and Pujol and Lavigne-Rebillard (1985) confirmed the existence of centrifugal nerves terminating in the human cochlea. Sacks and Lindenberg (1969) and Wolter (1991) reported that 5%–10% of the million-plus nerve fibers in the human optic nerve appear to be centrifugal fibers;[13] Briñón et al. (1998) reported that "abundant centrifugal fibers" appear to terminate in the human olfactory bulb (p. 3141); and Hans Spoendlin (1966) reported that 2% of the 30,000 cochlea-related fibers in the human vestibulo-cochlear nerve appear to be centrifugal fibers.

Physiological Findings

Physiological studies confirm that micro-electrode stimulation of the brain's visual, olfactory, and auditory pathways innervates the retina, the olfactory bulb, and the cochlea, respectively. Retinal activity has been modulated by electrically stimulating the visual pathway in cat brains (Granit, 1955; Hernández-Peón, Scherrer, & Velasco, 1956; Motokawa & Ebe, 1954), rat brains (Lörincz, Oláh, & Juhász, 2008), rabbit brains (Dodt, 1956), and monkey brains (Ogden & Brown, 1964), and by magnetically stimulating the visual cortex noninvasively in human brains (Gimranov, 2004). Olfactory-bulb activity has been modulated by electrically stimulating the olfactory pathway in cat brains (Hernández-Peón, Lavin, Alcocer-Cuarón, & Marcelin, 1960; Kerr & Hagbarth, 1955) and rat brains (Kunze, Shafton, Kemm, & McKenzie, 1991) and by optogenetically stimulating the olfactory pathway in mice brains (Ma & Luo, 2012). Cochlear activity has been modulated by electrically stimulating the auditory pathway in cat brains (Desmedt, 1962; Fex, 1959; Galambos, 1956), rat brains (Scates, Woods, & Azeredo, 1999), bat brains (Xiao & Suga, 2002), guinea pig brains (Mulders & Robertson, 2000), and human brains (Perrot et al., 2006).

Paralleling the above effects of CNS-stimulation on physiological responding "downstream" in the sensory receptors of warm-blooded animals, including humans, are the evocative effects of such stimulation on conscious sensation in humans. Micro-electrode stimulation of localized visual neurons in the human CNS sometimes innervates visual sensations (Lee, Hong, Seo, Tae, & Hong, 2000; Lozano et al., 1998; Penfield & Rasmussen, 1955). Transcranial magnetic stimulation of large areas in the visual cortex innervates phosphenes in most sighted persons (Elkin-Frankston, Fried, Pascual-Leone, Rushmore, & Valero-Cabr, 2010; Siniatchkin, Schlicke, & Stephani, 2011), but innervates phosphenes in only 20% of blind persons[14] (Théoret, Merabet, & Pascual-Leone, 2004), and innervates tactile sensations in many blind persons (Kupers et al., 2006; Ptito, Fumal, Schoenen, Gjedde, & Kupers, 2008). Micro-electrode stimulation of olfactory areas in the human CNS sometimes innervates olfactory sensations (Okun et al., 2007; Penfield & Rasmussen, 1955). Likewise, micro-electrode stimulation of auditory areas in the human CNS sometimes innervates auditory sensations (Bhatnagar, Andy, & Linville, 1989; Dostrovsky, Davis, Lee, Sher, & Tasker, 1993; Penfield & Rasmussen, 1955). And most interestingly, micro-electrode stimulation of somatosensory cortex in the human CNS innervates sensations of touch, just as *simultaneous* tactile stimulation of the skin innervates sensations of touch; but, to the surprise of many researchers, the tactile sensations stimulated by the electrical pulse on the skin emerge *one half second sooner* than the tactile sensations stimulated *simultaneously* by the micro-electrode in somatosensory cortex (Libet, Wright, Feinstein, & Pearl, 1979). Of course, this classic "problem of subjective timing" is surprising and problematic only if sensations of touch are assumed to be the subjective qualities of somatosensory cortex. It is a pseudoproblem, however, if sensations of touch are the subjective qualities of touch receptors in the skin and if micro-electrode stimulation of somatosensory cortex takes one half second to centrifugally innervate those touch receptors, in accordance with the evidence reviewed in this chapter.

It should be noted that, because the afferent signals from nociceptors are modulated by centrifugal fibers terminating in the spine instead of the pain receptors themselves (Millan, 2002), electrical stimulation of the human CNS does not normally innervate sensations of pain (Devor, 2007; Libet, 1973; Penfield & Rasmussen, 1955). Rather, CNS-stimulated pain tends to arise primarily in poststroke-pain patients who are electrically stimulated *above* their lesions and deafferentated nerves (Davis, Kiss, Tasker, & Dostrovsky, 1996; Katayama et al., 2001), So apparently, like the free nerve endings that we call nociceptors, deafferated nerve endings can be accompanied by the subjective quality of pain when they are corticofugally innervated or otherwise stimulated (Devor, 2009).

Psychophysiological Findings

Thus, the nervous system as it has evolved in warm-blooded animals appears to be equipped for the centrifugal construction of visually imaged sensations at the retinal level, odoriferously imaged sensations at the olfactory-bulb level, and auditorily imaged sensations at the cochlear level. As we shall see, presently available data indicate that both dreaming and wakeful imaging corticofugally affect activity within sensory transmitters, in particular activity within the retina, the cochlea, and the olfactory bulb.

Looking into retinal effects of the rapid-eye-movement dream state, Galambos, Szabó-Salfay, Szatmári, and Juhász (2001) found that the rat's retinal responsiveness during REM sleep can exhibit waking levels of responsiveness, slow-wave-sleep levels of responsiveness, and levels wavering in between. Given such findings, Galambos and his colleagues note that "two REM states are recognized in many animals, one with dreaming, the other without," and suggest that "the REM variability our experiments establish so securely is correlated with dreaming" (p. 2087). On the other hand, looking into Michel Jouvet's (1962, 1967) demonstrations that cochlear responsiveness during REM sleep also wavers between waking levels and slow-wave-sleep levels of responsiveness, Baust, Berlucchi, and Moruzzi (1964) discovered that movements in the "middle ear [muscle (MEM)] underlie the *peripheral* changes of the auditory input . . . during desynchronized sleep" (p. 671). Irvine and Webster (1972) confirmed that MEM movements during sleep mediate changes in cochlear responsiveness to evoking clicks at or above 80 dB, but found that neither movements of MEM nor stages of sleep affect cochlear responsiveness to evoking clicks at or below 55 dB. Finally, despite the latter researchers' inability to find MEM-free cochlear effects of REM sleep, Tsuno, Kashiwadani, and Mori (2008) were able to show that olfactory-bulb responsiveness during REM sleep wavers between waking levels of responsiveness and slow-wave-sleep levels of responsiveness, much like retinal responsiveness during REM sleep.

The above effects of REM sleep on the retina and the olfactory bulb constitute indirect support for Külpe's (1893/1895) position on the corticofugal construction of dreams and images and, as such, constitute a small piece of evidence in a much bigger evidentiary picture. So let us now turn our attention from the sleeping animal's REM-influenced sensory transmissions to the waking human's corticofugally imaged sensations.

When a flashing white light's physical intensity and subjective brightness increase, the human electroretinoretinogram (ERG)—in particular, the flash-triggered b-wave of the ERG—increases in amplitude (Armington, 1974). Bogoslovskii and Semenovskaya (1959) and Freedman and Ronchi (1964) documented increases in both the flash ERG's b-wave amplitude and the triggering flash's subjective brightness, when light flashes were presented at constant intensity in Maxwellian view but were accompanied by a conditioned stimulus that had repeatedly been paired with brighter flashes. Furthermore, Bittini and Ronchi (1958) and Mori and Ronchi (1960) documented the physical presence of ERG b-waves and the subjective experience of light flashes when actual light flashes were expected but were absent immediately following a conditional stimulus.

When green-filtered light is flashed onto the retina, the flash-triggered b-wave of the ERG is unimodal, but when red-filtered light is flashed onto the retina, the flash-triggered b-wave of the ERG is bimodal (Armington, 1974), as electroretinogram tracings illustrate on the left side of Figure 3. When three very vivid imagers in one of my own ERG studies viewed 5 green-filtered flashes at a 1-sec interflash interval but imaged the flashes appearing red instead of green, over 15% of the resulting ERG b-waves were bimodal instead of unimodal (Kunzendorf, 1984), as sample electroretinograms from all three imagers illustrate in the upper right quadrant of Figure 3. Conversely, when the same three vivid imagers viewed 5 red-filtered flashes at a 1-sec interflash interval but imaged the flashes appearing green instead of red, over 15% of the resulting ERG b-waves were unimodal instead of bimodal, as illustrated in the lower right quadrant of Figure 3. All three of these vivid imagers reported that their imaged sensations of color in this study were vivid enough to "block out" any perceived sensations of the flashing light's actual color, just as their normally imaged sensations are vivid enough to block out any perceptual background.[15] In contrast, when the four research participants with the least vivid visual imagery tried to image the green-filtered flashes appearing red, all of their ERG b-waves remained unimodal, and when these four nonvivid imagers tried to image the 5 red-filtered flashes appearing green, all of their ERG b-waves remained bimodal. Consequently, across the 20 participants in this research, there was a statistically significant –.60 correlation between their score on Marks' (1973) Vividness of Visual Imagery Questionnaire (wherein lower scores represent move vivid visual imagery) and their proportion of ERG b-waves with modes reflecting the imaged color rather than the viewed color.

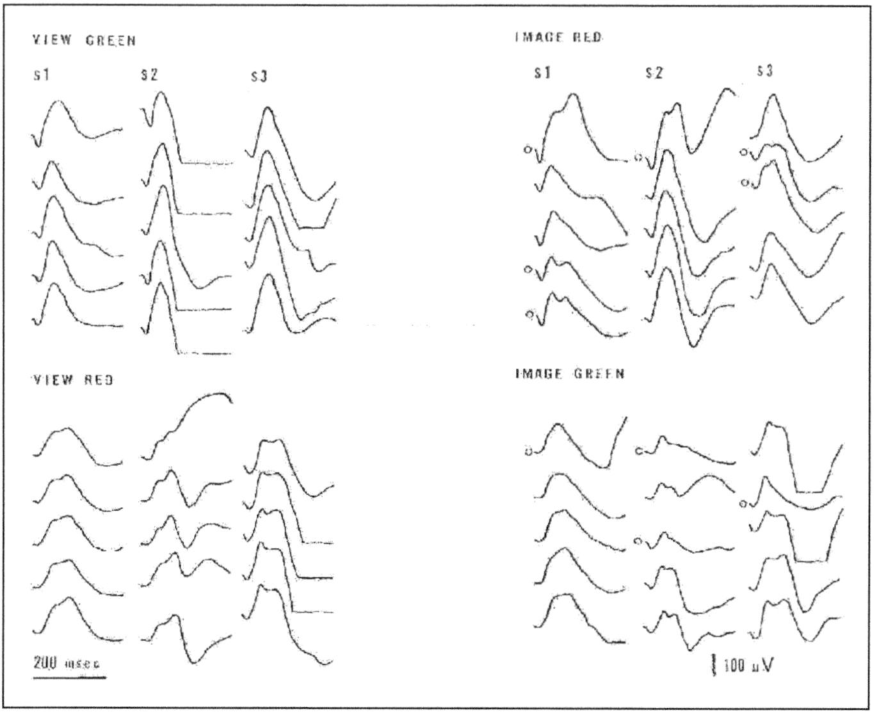

Figure 3. Tracings from Kunzendorf's (1984) data: three vivid imagers' electroretinographic responses to 5 green-filtered flashes which they viewed as such (upper left quadrant), to 5 red-filtered light flashes which they viewed as such (lower left quadrant), to 5 green-filtered light flashes which they imaged as red instead of green (upper right quadrant), and to 5 red-filtered light flashes which they imaged as green instead of red (lower right quadrant). The color-filtered flash ERGs that were judged to be complementary to the color of the flash are preceded by unfilled circles. Adapted from "Centrifugal Effects of Eidetic Imaging on Flash Electroretinograms and Autonomic Responses" by Robert G. Kunzendorf *Journal of Mental Imagery, 8*(4), 67-76. Copyright by Brandon House; reproduced with permission.

When the light-induced retinal fatigue preceding a flash ERG is increased, the ERG's b-wave amplitude is reduced (Armington, 1974). Kunzendorf and Hall (2001) demonstrated that, when imagery-induced retinal fatigue is increased prior to a flash, the flash's b-wave amplitude is similarly reduced. On imagery-induced-fatigue trials, the 66 research participants imaged a large bright light for 60 secs, stopped imaging and waited 5 secs, then viewed an ERG-initiating flash through an artificial pupil. On control trials, they waited 50 seconds, imaged a large bright light for 10 secs, stopped imaging and waited 5 secs, then viewed the ERG-initiating flash through the artificial pupil. For the 33 participants with more vivid imagery, b-wave amplitudes decreased significantly in the imagery-induced-fatigue condition, relative to the control condition; for the 33 participants with less vivid imagery, b-wave amplitudes did not decrease significantly in the imagery-induced-fatigue condition.

Given Doob's (1970) finding that 87% of children and 22% of adults experience visual images vivid enough to be "seen in front of" actual percepts, and given Kunzendorf's (1989) finding that 40% of children and 5% of adults generate visual images vivid enough to induce after-sensations of fixed retinal size, Kunzendorf, Justice, and Capone (1997) compared the electroretinographic effects of young children's imaging, their college-aged siblings' imaging, and art students' imaging. On randomly ordered control trials and "image brighter" trials, eight children, eight college-aged siblings of the children, and eight art students heard an 800 Hz beep for 750 msec, waited another 750 msecs, then viewed the ERG-initiating flash through an artificial pupil. Prior to beep onset on each control trial, instructions to "just look for a flash after the beep" were read aloud, and prior to beep onset on each "image brighter" trial, instructions to "after the beep, image a bright flash—brighter than any real flash" were read aloud. The b-wave amplitudes of the children's flash electroretinograms exhibited a significant 106% increase in the "image brighter" condition; the b-wave amplitudes of their college-aged siblings exhibited a nonsignificant 3% increase in the "image brighter" condition; and the b-wave amplitudes of the art students exhibited a significant 51% increase in the "image brighter" condition.

Measuring image-induced changes in the fMRI instead of the electroretinogram, Chen, Kato, Zhu, Ogawa, Tank, and Ugurbil (1998) found that visual imaging not only entails the centrifugal activation of primary visual cortex but also entails the corticofugal activation of lateral geniculate nuclei in some imagers. Notably, retinal ganglion cells extend from synaptic junctures in the lateral geniculate nuclei, all the way through the optic tract, into the retina itself (Pinel, 1997).

Other visual imaging research by D'Angiulli (2002) shows that image vividness increases with longer exposure to darkness or longer "dark adaptation," which increases the responsiveness of both rod cells and cone cells in the retina (Peachey, Arakawa, Alexander, & Marchese, 1992; Ruseckaite, Lamb, Pianta, & Cameron, 2011), but neither increases nor decreases the responsiveness of Area V1 in the visual cortex (Duffy & Hubel, 2007). Let us now turn our attention to imaged sensations other than visually imaged sensations.

Unlike above-cited investigations into the corticofugal construction of visual images at the retinal level, investigations into the corticofugal construction of smell images at the olfactory-bulb level have thus far been conducted only with mammals other than humans. In looking for centrifugally innervated olfactory-bulb patterns corresponding to the rabbit's olfactory "search images," Walter Freeman (1983) found that "changes in the [olfactory-bulb] EEG took place with changes in expectancy of odors and not merely with their presentation" (p. 1114). Kay and Freeman (1998) subsequently confirmed that, compared to the actual presentation of odors, the preafferent expectation of odors is associated with greater coherence between gamma oscillations in the olfactory bulb and gamma oscillations in the cortical origin of centrifugal fibers to the bulb.

Turning to the corticofugal construction of auditory images at the cochlear level, Kunzendorf, Jesses, Michaels, Caiazzo-Fluellen, and Butler (1991) examined the effects of auditory imaging on the brainstem auditory evoked potential (BSAEP)—a 10-msec-long potential that was repeatedly evoked by a .25-msec click at 55 dB and 8000 Hz and then was computer-averaged across 500 clicks separated by an interclick interval of 200-msecs. Specifically, my student co-authors and I examined the effects of imaging on the BSAEP's most prominent waveform—Wave 5, which originates in the inferior colliculus one synapse away from the cochlea, and which exhibits a shorter latency and larger amplitude when clicks are actually louder (Hughes, 1985; Picton, Hillyard, Krausz, & Galambos, 1974). My co-authors and I found that Wave 5's latency became significantly shorter when the 13 young children in the study imaged louder clicks, became significantly longer when the 13 music students in the study imaged softer clicks, and did not change when the 13 college-aged siblings of the children imaged louder or softer clicks. In addition, Wave 5's amplitude became significantly larger when the 13 young children imaged louder clicks. In a follow-up study, Kunzendorf and Boisvert (1996) found that Wave 5's amplitude became significantly larger when louder clicks were imaged by four research participants reporting very vivid imagery on the Vividness of Auditory Imagery Questionnaire (Kunzendorf, 1980, App. G) but not when louder clicks were imaged by four participants reporting less vivid auditory imagery. Also in the follow-up study, Wave 5's amplitude became significantly smaller when loud music drowning out the clicks was imaged by the four vivid imagers, but not when such music was imaged by the four participants with less vivid auditory imagery. It is not likely that these effects of auditory imaging on Wave 5 were mediated by imaging-induced contractions of the middle ear muscle, given that such contractions do not affect brainstem potentials that are evoked by tones as soft as 55 dB or as high as 8000 Hz (Irvine & Webster, 1972; Lukas, 1980, 1981).

THE FUNCTION OF VIVIDLY IMAGED, CENTRIFUGALLY CONSTRUCTED SENSATIONS

Psychology's 100-year-old quest to understand vivid imagery's functions is given new direction by the above findings of more vivid imagery in children and in artistic adults, as well as recent findings concerning the functions served by centrifugal control of the sensory transmitters in warm-blooded animals. Prior to the 21st century, empirical investigations into the function of vivid imaging received direction primarily from the autobiographical reports of scientists and artists who experienced either vivid imagery or dream imagery while resolving issues of interest to them (Barrett, 2001; Miller, 1986; Shepard, 1978). But contrary to empirical predictions based on such autobiographical reports, 20th century studies continually found vividness of visual imagery to be uncorrelated with measures of visual reasoning—specifically, with tests of geometrical problem solving (Betts, 1909; Bowers, 1935; Kunzendorf, 1982; Wood & Bell, 1920), with map reading exercises (Kunzendorf & Buker, 2008–2009; Poltrock & Brown, 1984), with measures of mental rotation (Ashton, McFarland, Walsh, & White, 1978; Dean & Morris, 1991; Hatakeyama, 1981; Kosslyn, Brunn, Cave, & Wallach, 1984; Logie, Pernet, Buonocore, & Della Sala, 2011; McKelvie & Rohrberg, 1978; Poltrock & Brown, 1984), with mental paper-folding exercises (Bethel-Fox, Lohman, & Snow, 1984; Dean & Morris, 1991; DiVesta, Ingersoll, & Sunshine, 1971; Durndell & Wetherick, 1976; Lorenz & Neisser, 1985; McKelvie & Rohrberg, 1978; Poltrock & Brown, 1984; Richardson, 1977), with tests of directed mental synthesis (Antonietti, Bologna, & Lupi, 1997; Kunzendorf, Young, Beecy, & Beals, 2000; Morrison & Wallace, 2001), with mental cube-cutting exercises (Kunzendorf et al., 2000; Parrott, 1986; Poltrock & Brown, 1984; Wood & Bell, 1920) and, according to McKelvie's (1995) meta-analysis of published studies, with visual creativity measures overall. The early 20th century evidence indicating that the astuteness of people's visuo-spatial reasoning does not depend on the vividness of their visual imagery led John Watson (1913) to write off subjectively experienced images as epiphenomena with no causal effects on behavior. And toward the end of the 20th century, the accrued findings of no dependency led Stephen Kosslyn (1994) to redefine the mental image so as to "refer to the internal representation that is used in information processing, not the experience itself" (p. 3). But according to Külpe's (1893/1895) argument for the corticofugal construction of visually imaged sensations from imageless thought, the astuteness of such thought cannot possibly depend on the vividness of any visually imaged sensations afterwards constructed from it. Only imageless cortical thinking that requires the corticofugal innervation of sensory receptors should, on Külpe's account, be dependent on (i.e., correlated with) greater vividness of visually imaged sensations.

The latter account—in conjunction with the above findings of retinopetal innervation during children's and artists' visual imaging, as well as the following findings of retinopetal innervation during warm-blooded animals' rule development—raises the interesting possibility that individual differences in vividly imaged, centrifugally innervated sensations might actually be developmental differences related both to the acquisition of sensory-motor rules in young warm-blooded animals and to the refinement of such rules in human artists. So presently, let us consider the data suggesting that corticofugal control of the sensory receptors plays a role in the process of rule development in warm-blooded animals; then let us consider the theory and the data suggesting that the construction of vivid sensory images plays a beneficial role in the process of rule development in human beings.

It turns out that the particular processes that centrifugally innervate the retina, the olfactory bulb, and the cochlea differ across species, dramatically so across warm-blooded and cold-blooded animals, because the underlying centrifugal pathways in different animals originate in different brain areas (Fujita, Satou, & Ueda, 1984; Repérant et al., 2006; Roberts & Meredith, 1992). In fish, efferent retinal nerves originate in the olfactory nervous system and increase retinal responsiveness during olfactory stimulation (Maaswinkel & Li, 2003; Weiss & Meyer, 1988); in birds, efferent retinal nerves are thought to be part of feedback circuits embodying the sensory-motor schemata for selecting and pecking food (Hahmann & Güntürkün, 1992); in mammals, including human beings, efferent retinal nerves' "functional role . . . is far from having been resolved" (Repérant et al., 2006, p. 39).[16] Efferent olfactory nerves in fish interact with trigeminal nerves and allow for tactile and thermal modulation of the olfactory bulb (Belousova, Devitsina, & Malyukina, 1983); efferent olfactory nerves in birds influence olfactory navigation (Patzke, Manns, & Güntürkün, 2011); and efferent olfactory nerves in mammals play a role in odor-discrimination rule-learning (Cohen, Reuveni, Barkai, & Maroun, 2008). Efferent cochlear nerves in fish are comingled with efferent vestibular nerves and are conjointly involved in postural orientation (Platt, 1973); efferent cochlear nerves in birds are positioned adjacent to efferent vestibular nerves and are thought to be involved in sensory-motor rule-development for birdsong (Wild, Krützfeldt, & Kubke, 2010; Williams, 1989); efferent cochlear nerves in mammals are separated from efferent vestibular nerves, are projected in tonotopic correspondence with the tone-specific cortical cells from which they originate (Lim & Anderson, 2007), and appear to be involved in the development of sensory-motor timing rules (Ohlrogge, Doucet, & Ryugo, 2001; Suga, Ziao, Ma, & Ji, 2002), including timing rules for the human perception of speech (Veuillet, Magnan, Ecalle, Thai-Van, & Collet, 2007). Thus, in cold-blooded animals like the species of fish studied to date, the centrifugal pathways to sensory receptors in a particular modality tend to originate in other sensory systems and tend to play a role in modulating the receptors in that particular modality. In warm-blooded animals like the species of birds and mammals in the above studies, on the other hand, centrifugal pathways to sensory receptors in a particular modality tend to originate in cortical areas and tend to play a role in the development of sensory-motor rules for that particular modality.

Theoretically, the cognitive process by which warm-blooded animals develop sensory-motor rules represents an evolutionary advancement over the process by which warm- and cold-blooded animals learn stimulus-response associations. The rules that develop in the warm-blooded animal's cortex can appropriately parse afferent input never encountered before and can appropriately generate efferent output never required before. In contrast, the associations that form in both the warm-blooded animal's and cold-blooded animal's brain apply only to stimuli empirically encountered before and account only for responses actually generated before. The process of associative learning is easy for us to understand. But in order for us to understand how the mind develops rules that are neither ingrained innately in the brain nor experienced empirically through the senses, we must acquaint ourselves with the developmental psychologist Jean Piaget's (1970) thesis: that schemata or imageless sensory-motor rules are creatively hypothesized in the child's mind, are subsequently tested to determine whether they adequately assimilate conscious sensations, are thereafter accommodated or revised as necessary, are then retested and refined, and so on. With regard to the role played by centrifugally imaged sensations in this developmental process of hypothesizing, testing, and refining rules, Kunzendorf (1990) suggested that vividly imaged sensations are corticofugally generated from the developing "grammatical rules" for parsing perceptual sensations into imageless cortical percepts and are compared against concurrently perceived or remembered sensations in order to test the developing rules' adequacy and to guide their refinement. According to this suggestion, cortically hypothesized rules guide the centrifugal generation of retinal "test images" during the development of "visual grammar" and guide the centripetal parsing of retinal input following grammar development, just as cortically hypothesized rules guide the centrifugal generation of babbled sentences during the development of linguistic grammar and guide the centripetal parsing of linguistic input following grammar development. Thus, while the rules of visual grammar are being developed, children sometimes generate mental images and paper-and-pencil drawings of roundish houses (Cox, 2005) and misaligned human figures (Goodnow & Friedman, 1972), and such "test images" and underdeveloped drawings serve as corrective feedback for further grammatical development and future rule refinement. Consistent with the current suggestion, three 21st century studies have demonstrated that the ability to image vividly is positively correlated with the ability to hypothesize, test, and refine new rules, even though it was not correlated with the ability to apply old rules to new problem sets in 20th century research.

In the first of these three studies, Kunzendorf and Reynolds (2004–2005) examined the correlation between the ability to develop rules of topological equivalence (across two conditions of instruction) and the ability to image vividly. The 30 participants in the study's "visual imaging" condition were instructed as follows:

> In this experiment, your mind will be developing the rules of topology much the same way that, in early childhood, your mind developed the rules of linear perspective. The rules of linear perspective capture the transformation of visual appearances as we move about in the world. Thus, even though a car appears smaller after it has moved away from us, we consider it to be equivalent to the car we saw before, because the rules of linear perspective capture this size transformation. Topology, a branch of mathematics, provides a different set of rules for transforming visual appearances in a manner that we have not previously experienced. On each trial in this experiment, you will be presented with three figures, two of which are

> topologically equivalent. On some trials, you will be told which of the three figures are topologically equivalent, and on other trials, you will have to decide for yourself which two figures are topologically equivalent. On all trials, you should actively try to figure out the rules that define topologically equivalent figures. The best way to figure out these rules is to use your visual imagination, as children use theirs, to try visually to transform one figure into another—to try out various transformational rules through trial-and-error visualizing, in other words. When children develop the rules of linear perspective, they test many possible rules of size transformation through playful trial-and-error visualizing (rather than formal logic or verbal thinking). So, throughout this experiment, let your mind develop an intuitive visual understanding of the rules of topology, by engaging in some trial-and-error visualizing of possible transformational rules.

In the study's control condition, instructions to 30 more participants omitted the final two sentences above and ended with the sentence, "On all trials, you should actively try to figure out the rules that define topologically equivalent figures, *by whatever method or strategy that works best for you.*" The participants needed to figure out that topologically equivalent figures can be rotated and stretched and twisted until they match, but cannot be cut and pasted in order to match, as the sample test trial in Figure 4 allows us to appreciate. Across all 16 of the study's actual test trials, participants who received imaging instructions correctly identified significantly more of the topologically equivalent figures than participants in the control condition did. And controlling for the conditions of instruction, the likelihood of correctly identifying the topologically equivalent figures correlated significantly with greater image vividness on the Vividness of Vividness of Visual Imagery Questionnaire. Thus, this first study's findings

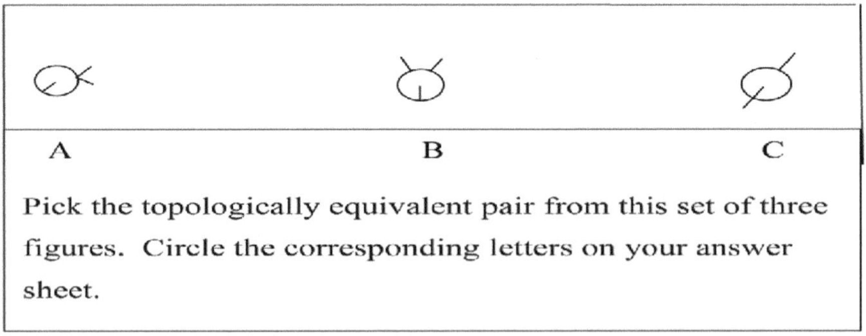

Figure 4. Sample test trial on which the topological equivalence of A and C is tested. Adapted from "On the Cognitive Function of Visual Images and the Development of Individual Differences" by R. G. Kunzendorf and K. Reynolds (2004–2005). Reproduced with permission.

provided initial evidence consistent with the thesis that vividly imaged sensations foster the testing and refinement of newly developing rules.

In the second study, Kunzendorf and Buker (2008–2009) examined correlations between the ability to develop rules of linear perspective—either the not-yet-developed rules of 3-point "bird's eye" perspective (3PP), or the already-developed rules of 2-point "ground level" perspective (2PP)—and the ability to construct vivid visual images. The 112 participants in the "bird's-eye perspective" condition received 20 test trials that were variations on the test trial depicted in Figure 5 and were followed by study trials with corrective feedback; the 116 participants in the "ground-level perspective" condition received 20 test trials that were variations on the test trial depicted in Figure 6 and were also followed by study trials with corrective feedback. On all test trials, the participants in both conditions received instructions asking them to identify how the target would look from the same viewing distance but from a different perspective; and on all study trials, the participants in both conditions received corrective

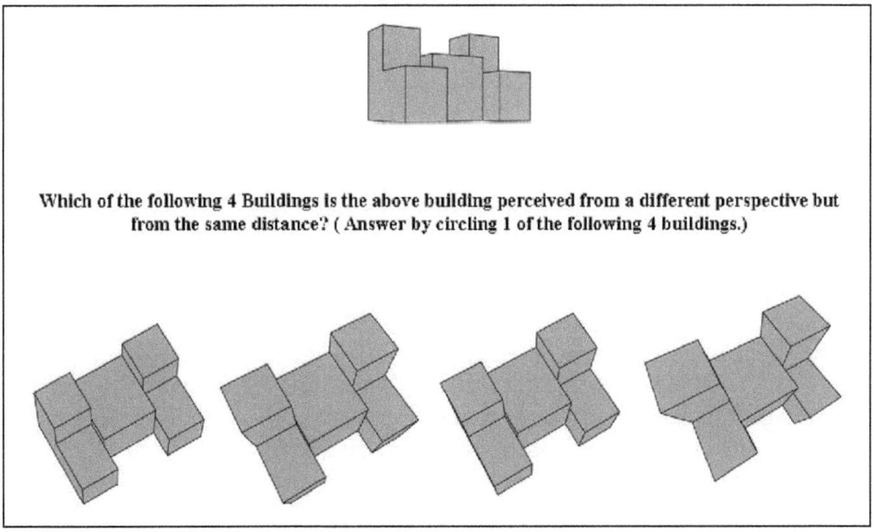

Figure 5. Three-point-perspective condition's third test-slide, depicting four test structures from a viewing orbit 70º above a ground-level fulcrum on the target structure's floor. (The second test-structure from the right has the target's "angle of view" or viewing distance.) Adapted from "Should Visual Images be Defined as Depictive Neural Patterns, or as Conscious Sensations Constructed from 'Imageless' Visual Thoughts?" by R. G. Kunzendorf and F. Buker (2008–2009). Reproduced with permission.

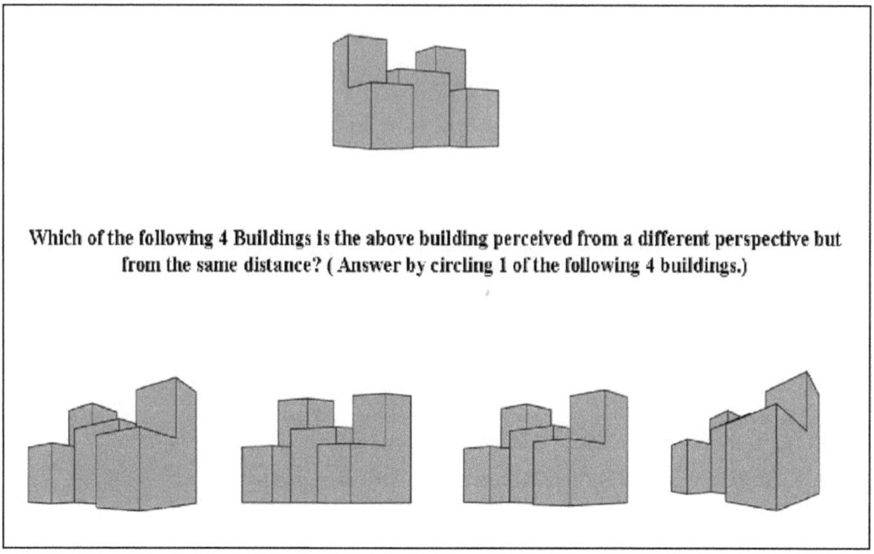

Figure 6. Two-point-perspective condition's third test-slide, depicting four test structures from ground-level viewpoints 70° counter-clockwise from the target structure's viewpoint. (The second test-structure from the right has the target's "angle of view" or viewing distance.) Adapted from "Should Visual Images Be Defined as Depictive Neural Patterns, or as Conscious Sensations Constructed From 'Imageless' Visual Thoughts?" by R. G. Kunzendorf and F. Buker (2008–2009). Reproduced with permission.

feedback containing the right answer, plus the following instruction: "In order to develop the underlying transformational rules, use your visual imagination to transform the figures and test out different rules." In the "bird's eye" condition, the early-trial likelihood of already knowing 3PP rules was not high and not correlated with image vividness, but the late-trial improvement in 3PP knowledge was significant in itself and was significantly correlated with greater image vividness on the Vividness of Visual Imagery Questionnaire. In the "ground level" condition, the early-trial likelihood of already knowing 2PP rules was relatively high but was not correlated with image vividness; and the late-trial improvement in 2PP knowledge was not significant in itself and was not correlated with greater image vividness. This finding that image vividness correlates significantly with 3PP rule development, but not with 2PP rule application, provides support for another implication of the current thesis: that vividly imaged sensations facilitate the testing and refinement of any newly developing rule from which they are constructed, but not the application of any sensation-parsing rule already tested and refined.

In the third study, Kunzendorf et al. (2012–2013) examined the correlation of visual imaging ability with the ability to develop visuo-spatial 3PP rules, as in Kunzendorf and Buker's (2008–2009) study, and the correlation of auditory imaging ability with the ability to develop Reber and Allen's (1978) audio-temporal grammar for differentiating rule-compliant and rule-defiant sequences of tones. In the study's experimental condition for visuo-spatial rule development, twenty 3PP test trials similar to the sample trial in Figure 5 were alternated with study trials giving participants corrective feedback and instructing them to use their "visual imagination to transform the figures and test out different rules." In the study's experimental condition for audio-temporal rule development, each of 24 test trials presented 14 tonal patterns in succession—five exemplary patterns governed by grammatical rules, two test patterns (one grammatical pattern and one nongrammatical pattern), the same five exemplary patterns, then the same two test patterns—and instructed participants to identify which of the two test patterns was grammatical. Alternating with these 24 test trials were study trials, which presented all 14 tonal patterns again (along with corrective visual feedback for test patterns) and which instructed participants to use auditory imagery, while listening, to anticipate grammatical tones in their mind's ear. Across 83 participants in the visuo-spatial rule-development condition, greater development of 3PP rules correlated significantly with greater vividness of visual imagery, but not auditory imagery. Conversely, across 94 participants in audio-temporal rule-development condition, greater development of grammatical rules correlated significantly with greater vividness of auditory imagery, but not visual imagery. Such modality-specific correlations between imageless visuo-spatial rules and vivid visual images, and between imageless audio-temporal rules and vivid auditory images, are consistent with still another implication of the current thesis: that the specific cortical rules of imageless thoughts from which vividly imaged sensations are constructed, and the vividly imaged sensations themselves, are interconnected, presumably by modality-specific corticofugal pathways.

On this account, the reason why most adults image less vividly than they did during early childhood is because they no longer need to develop new sensorial-perceptual rules and therefore no longer need to corticofugally generate vivid test images at the level of the sensory transmitter— unless they are artists or musicians or otherwise creative persons who are continually refining their sensorial-perceptual rules. After developing basic sensorial-perceptual rules, people still need to develop cognitive and social and cultural rules. But in order to test rules of the latter sort, they need only construct "a sketchy image," which minimizes the number of sensations necessary to maintain "structural relations" and which subjectively seems "faint to the extent of being barely observable" (Arnheim, 1969, pp. 109–115). Thus, without regard to the vividness of people's imagery, Jerome Singer (1994) details how people generate images to test the cognitive rules guiding their thought about "possible futures" and "alternative courses of action" (p. 7); Eric Klinger (1992) details how people generate images to test the cognitive and social rules circumscribing their pursuit of goals; James Honeycutt (2008) details how people generate "imagined interactions" to test the social rules governing their interpersonal behavior; Sheikh and Sheikh (2003) detail how people generate images to test the cultural rules defining their scheme for coping with human mortality; Ernest Hartmann (1995) details how people generate dream images to picture their emotions and to test schemes for coping with those emotions; and Deirdre Barrett (2001) and Roger Shepard (1978) detail how people generate dream images to test a variety of newly hypothesized rules. Furthermore, in research suggesting that dream images in nonhuman animals can play a similar rule-testing function, Gupta, van der Meer, Touretzky, and Redish (2010) found that the microelectrode-measured "cognitive maps" within the brains of maze-trained rats tend, during REM sleep (i.e., dreaming), to become innervated not only along recently learned pathways in those neuro-cognitive maps but also along nonnavigated shortcuts in those maps.

THE EVOLUTION OF RULE DEVELOPMENT IN WARM-BLOODED ANIMALS

Noam Chomsky (1968) asserted that the development of hierarchical sequencing rules is unique to human brains and that the learning of associations is ubiquitous across animal nervous systems. As Chomsky famously demonstrated, hierarchical sequencing rules allow us to *parse* temporally sequenced but hierarchically organized input—for example, the hierarchically structured sentence, "The trustee who admonished the Penn State administrators who protected the football coach who abused boys who needed a father figure was red-faced," a sentence structure that is both novel and grammatical, albeit memory-taxing, because it has four recursively embedded clauses within it. If our minds could do no more than associate the contiguous elements within sentences, then we would have no way of knowing that the "trustee" (the first noun in above sentence) "was red-faced" and the "father figure" (the noun contiguous to the verb phrase) was not. In addition to allowing us to parse input, hierarchical sequencing rules allow us to *generate* temporally sequenced but hierarchically organized output such as the "Penn State" sentence above, whereas associations by continuity allow us only to piece together contiguously associated word classes into a sentence structure that is not likely to be grammatical if it is novel and is not likely to be novel if it is grammatical.

Consistent with Chomsky's (1968) assertion that the learning of associations is ubiquitous across animal species, studies have documented associative learning not only in warm-blooded animals, but also in fish (Bull, 1928, 1935; Washburn & Bentley, 1906), in insects (Byrne & Crow, 1991; Giurfa & Sandoz, 2012), and in molluscs (Byrne & Crow, 1991; Neary, Crow, & Alkon, 1981). But contrary to Chomsky's assertion that the development of hierarchical sequencing rules is unique to human beings, research requiring warm-blooded animals to discriminate rule-governed temporal sequences from rule-violating temporal sequences has shown that rats can develop the sequencing rules behind hierarchically organized inputs (Fountain, 2008), that dolphins can develop the sequencing rules in an artificial grammar (Herman, Richards, & Wolz, 1984; Schusterman & Gisiner, 1988), and that birds can develop the sequencing rules behind recursively structured inputs (Gentner, Fenn, Margoliash, & Nusbaum, 2006) as well as the sequencing rules in an artificial grammar (Herbranson & Shimp, 2003, 2008).

Interestingly, Reber and Allen (1978, 2000) assert that the rules of artificial grammars are developed implicitly rather than consciously, and fMRI studies show that the development of artificial grammars is statistically associated with active engagement of the prefrontal cortex in humans (Fletcher, Büchel, Josephs, Friston, & Dolan, 1999; Strange, Henson, Friston, & Dolan, 2001)—consistent with the supposition in Chapter 2 that all cortical knowledge is implicit or sensationless. And as earlier sections of this chapter indicate, development of the sequencing rules in such grammars is statistically associated both with greater vividness of auditory imaging in humans (Kunzendorf et al., 2012–2013) and with greater centrifugal innervation of the cochlea in humans (Veuillet et al., 2007). Plus, development of the sequencing rules in the audio-temporal "grammars" of bats, rats, and birds has been statistically associated with centrifugal innervation of the cochlea as well (Ohlrogge et al., 2001; Suga et al., 2002; Wild et al., 2010; Williams, 1989). All of these statistical associations are consistent with the current chapter's thesis regarding auditorily imaged sensations at the cochlear level: that, as warm-blooded animals develop sensationless cortical rules for the perceptual parsing of cochlear sensations, they may corticofugally generate rule-governed "test images" containing cochlear sensations.

Of course, sequencing rules for parsing temporal input and for generating temporal output aren't the only rules that warm-blooded animals can develop. Interspatial rules for parsing visual input from aerial perspectives and for guiding motoric output during aerial navigation are developed by birds (Jones, Antoniadis, Shettleworth, & Kamil, 2002; Spetch, Rust, Kamil, & Jones, 2003); plus, interspatial rules for parsing "bird's eye" input and for generating "bird's eye" images can be developed by humans with vivid visual imagery (Kunzendorf & Buker, 2008–2009; Kunzendorf et al., 2012–2013). And like the development of sequencing rules, the development of interspatial rules and visuo-motor schemas is statistically associated with active engagement of the prefrontal cortex in humans (Lee et al., 2012), in monkeys (Goodwin, Blackman, Sakellaridi, & Chafee, 2012; Ryou & Wilson, 2004), and in rats (Rossetti & Carboni, 2005), and is associated with corticofugal innervation of the retina in birds (Hahmann & Güntürkün, 1992). These statistical associations are consistent with the current thesis regarding visually imaged sensations at the retinal level: that, as warm-blooded animals develop sensationless cortical rules for the perceptual parsing of retinal sensations, they may corticofugally generate rule-governed "test images" containing retinal sensations.

EPILOGUE: THE PHYSICAL BRAINS AND THE MENTAL IMAGES OF WARM-BLOODED ANIMALS

The mammal's prefrontal cortex and the bird's forebrain equivalent—the nidopallium caudolaterale, which many researchers nominally identify as prefrontal cortex—serve to distinguish warm-blooded animals from cold-blooded animals (Güntürkün, 2005, 2012; Mogensen & Divac, 1982; Reiner, 1986). Indeed, the evolution of prefrontal cortex is the primary reason why warm-blooded species' brain weights, relative to their body weights, is a "quantum leap" higher than cold-blooded species' relative brain weights. This evolutionary discontinuity between warm-blooded brains and cold-blooded brains is dramatically illustrated in Figure 7's reproduction of Harry Jerison's (1985) graph. For 623 vertebrate species, Jerison determined the ratio of log brain

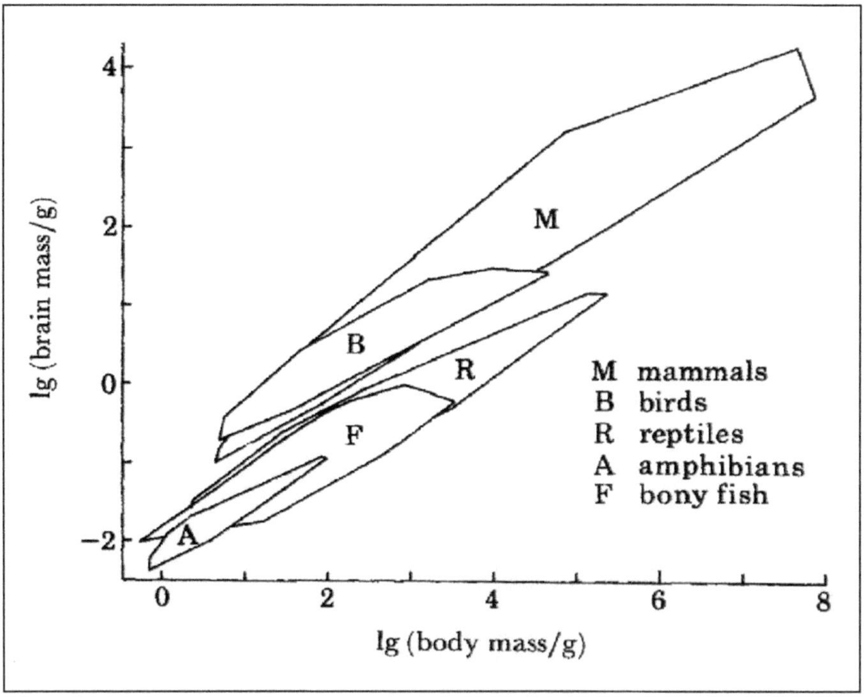

Figure 7. Brain-body relations in living species from five vertebrate classes: mammals and birds (Martin, 1981; 309 species of placental mammals and 180 species of birds), bony fish (Ridet, 1973; 46 species), amphibians (Thireau, 1975; 40 species), and reptiles (Platel, 1979; 48 species). The polygons are minimum convex hulls drawn about the data of each class. Adapted from "Animal Intelligence as Encephalization" by H. J. Jerison (1985). Reproduced with permission.

mass over log body mass, then drew a best-fitting polygon around the 309 mammalian ratios, a second polygon around the 180 avian ratios, a third polygon around the 48 reptilian ratios, a fourth polygon around the 40 amphibian ratios, and a fifth polygon around the 46 ratios for bony fish. As Figure 7 indicates, the polygons for warm-blooded vertebrates—mammals and birds—are a "quantum leap" higher than the polygons for cold-blooded vertebrates.

This chapter commenced with one qualitative difference between warm-blooded and cold-blooded animals—the evolution of REM sleep and dreaming in mammals and birds—and concludes with another qualitative difference between warm-blooded and cold-blooded animals—the evolution of prefrontal cortex in mammals and birds. Connecting dream imagery and prefrontal cortex, along with the evidentiary threads in between, is this chapter's evolutionary thesis: that, while the rules for anticipating and parsing perceptual sensations are being developed in prefrontal cortex, vividly imaged sensations tend to be corticofugally constructed at the sensory-receptor level in order to test the developing schema or developing set of rules.

As neuroscientist Joaquín Fuster (2000) notes, the function of prefrontal cortex's "*executive* memory" (also called *working* memory) is to develop anticipatory sensory-motor rules, not to execute old schemes:

> This kind of memory probably consists of widely distributed neuronal networks representing schemes of temporally organized action in the form of general plans, procedures, or programs of behavior. Included are complex schemes of behavior that have been recently acquired. The qualifications of novelty and complexity are important, because, after it has been firmly consolidated, automatic or routine behavior appears represented and enacted by neural structures at lower stages of the motor hierarchy. (p. 128)
>
> Its role is to prepare the motor apparatus for anticipated actions and sensory receptors for sensory signals releasing or accompanying those actions. The setting of effectors and receptors for prospective actions is the temporal mirror image of active short-term memory. Instead of recent memory, this is "memory for the future." (Ingvar, 1985)

And as psychological scientist David Geary (2009) notes, schematic rules that develop in the prefrontal cortices of mammals and birds—unlike simple associations that develop in the brains of all vertebrates—are "important for self-awareness, awareness of one's behavior in social contexts, and the ability to anticipate future events" (pp. 24–26). So now let us turn our attention to the evolution of self-awareness in certain warm-blooded animals—specifically, those birds and mammals requiring 2 or more years to reach sexual maturity—and let us consider the survival advantage that self-awareness confers on such birds and mammals.

CHAPTER 4

The Evolution of Consciousness of Self

> In many discussions of the problem of consciousness, the word *consciousness* seems to refer to something more like *self-consciousness.* These discussions are concerned not with a simple, first-order awareness—whether of sensations, images, objects, qualities, events, or thoughts—but with some kind of second-order awareness of oneself as a conscious agent [or subject] distinct from the nonself or of the fact of one's first-order awareness. In contrast to simpler and more direct consciousness in the first two senses, second-order awareness may have emerged only relatively recently in primate evolution.
>
> —"On the Physical Basis, Linguistic Representation, and Conscious Experience of Colors," Roger N. Shepard (1993, p. 232)

This fourth and final chapter develops the thesis that self-consciousness—manifested either as self-consciousness that *one is imaging sensations* or as self-consciousness that *one is perceiving sensations*—tends to promote survival and to evolve in warm-blooded animals whose cortical rules are hypothesized, *imaginally tested*, and refined over a pre-adulthood period of 2 or more years. But before we can meaningfully discuss the evolution of self-consciousness or awareness of "self as subject," we must differentiate it from self-concept or awareness of "self as object" and from self-efficacy or awareness of "self as agent." So let us begin by considering how these three types of self-awareness are theoretically defined in this chapter and how they are scientifically measured in the research literature. Thereafter, let us focus on the particular mammals and birds whose behaviors indicate that they possess a self-concept and, by implication, self-consciousness. And finally, as this chapter and this book draw to a close, let us turn our attention to the wakeful deactivation of self-conscious source verification in some psychologically distressed persons, but not in other distressed persons, and let us contemplate the implications for future human evolution.

DEFINING AND MEASURING THE ILLUSORY SELF-CONSCIOUS EXPERIENCE OF "SELF AS SUBJECT"

When Gottfried Leibniz (1765/1896) rejected the Cartesian position that a soul or immaterial "subject of consciousness" is implicitly *conscious of* itself being *conscious of* physical "objects of consciousness," he posited instead that some neural states are paralleled by conscious sensations, other neural states by an illusory experience of "self as subject," and that conscious sensations are sometimes accompanied by this experience of self-consciousness, other times not. During normal dreaming, for example, the visual sensations experienced in one's dream are not accompanied by one's waking sense of self-consciousness that *one is having the experience*, not unless one wakes up with the sensations still in mind and then experiences one's waking sense of self-consciousness in relation to those sensations. Thus, as Morton Prince (1910) noted,

> Whether we are self-conscious of any given state of consciousness must depend, it would seem, upon whether the brain process, correlated with it, is synthesized in a particular way with the larger system of brain processes which is correlated at a given moment with the self-conscious. . . . And in so far as a brain process can occur detached from the main system of processes, so far can consciousness occur without self-consciousness. (p. 94)

Where Leibniz's and Prince's positions on self-consciousness fall short, however, is in not explicating how the experience of "self as subject" might have evolved—how it might have been naturally selected to perform a function more adaptive than simply imparting to us the illusion of "having" our sensory experiences. This shortcoming has recently been remedied by source-verification theory's functional understanding of the self-conscious experience of "self as subject."

The illusory sense of oneself as a *subject of consciousness* who either knowingly "has" sensations or is "conscious of" sensory objects, according to Kunzendorf's (1987–1988, 2000, 2010) source-verification theory, is a generic manifestation of either the tacit knowledge that *one is imaging sensations* or the tacit knowledge that *one is perceiving sensations*. The tacit self-awareness that *one is imaging certain visual sensations*, on Kunzendorf's account, is the subjective aspect of a neural process that is actively registering the corticofugal innervation of the retinal substrate of those visual sensations. Conversely, the tacit self-awareness that *one is perceiving particular sensations* is the subjective aspect of the same source-verification process when it is instead registering the peripheral innervation of the retinal substrate of the latter sensations. The neural source-verification process itself is not "conscious of" the sensations paralleling the retinal substrates that it is physically registering. Rather, the tacit self-awareness that *one is imaging* or *perceiving*, in relation to particular sensations, is the subjective aspect of this neural process so long as it is operative and is neither asleep nor otherwise rendered inoperative.

Scientific evidence that such a source-verification process is indeed operative during normal wakefulness in normal humans comes from an experimental paradigm employed in a half-dozen studies conducted by Kunzendorf and his students (Kunzendorf, 1980, 1985–1986a; Kunzendorf et al., 1996–1997; Kunzendorf & Hall, 2001; Kunzendorf & Karpen, 1996–1997; Kunzendorf, Moran, et al., 1995–1996). In all of these studies, research participants on each of many trials perceived a visual stimulus on one side of a fixation point and mentally imaged the same visual stimulus on the other side of the fixation point, then rated the vividness of the trial's mental image from "0 = no image" to "5 = as vivid and clear as the actual stimulus." Thereafter, while continuing to image and perceive the trial's stimulus, the participants were signaled to identify the side with the image or the side with the percept as quickly and as accurately as possible. For each participant, the best-fitting slope of his or her image-identification times over his or her vividness ratings was computed. As Figure 8 illustrates, this within-subject slope for normal subjects during normal wakefulness tended to be, paradoxically, a negative slope, indicating that perceived sensations were discriminated more quickly from vividly imaged sensations introspectively similar to the perceived sensations, and more slowly from faintly imaged sensations introspectively different from the perceived sensations.

Kunzendorf's (1987–1988, 2000, 2010) source-verification theory is able to make sense of this paradox by theorizing (a) that vividly imaged sensations require greater corticofugal innervation of the retina and (b) that greater corticofugal innervation can be more quickly registered by the nervous system's source-verification process (so long as the process is operative).[17] At the same time, source-verification theory is able to make sense of the positive within-subject slopes obtained for hypnotized subjects (Kunzendorf, 1985–1986a), psychosis-prone subjects (Kunzendorf, Moran et al., 1995–1996), dissociation-prone subjects (Kunzendorf & Karpen, 1996–1997), and psychosomatic imagers (Kunzendorf et al., 1996–1997) by positing that hypnotic, psychotic, and dissociative states, like normal states of sleep, deactivate the nervous system's source-verification process.

Similarities and differences between the psychotic and the dissociative deactivation of self-conscious source-verifying will be addressed later in this chapter. The many effects of hypnotically deactivated source-verification—effects on spontaneous and suggested hallucinating, on dissociated perceiving with or without Ernest Hilgard's (1977) "hidden observer," on spontaneous and irreversible "posthypnotic amnesia" for the source of sensations, on hypnotic hypermnesia for subliminally stimulated percepts, and on the hypnotic recovery of dissociated memories and the hypnotic creation of false memories—have been reviewed by Kunzendorf (2010) and will not be reviewed again in this chapter, as they fall outside the evolutionary focus of this book. The effect of failing to

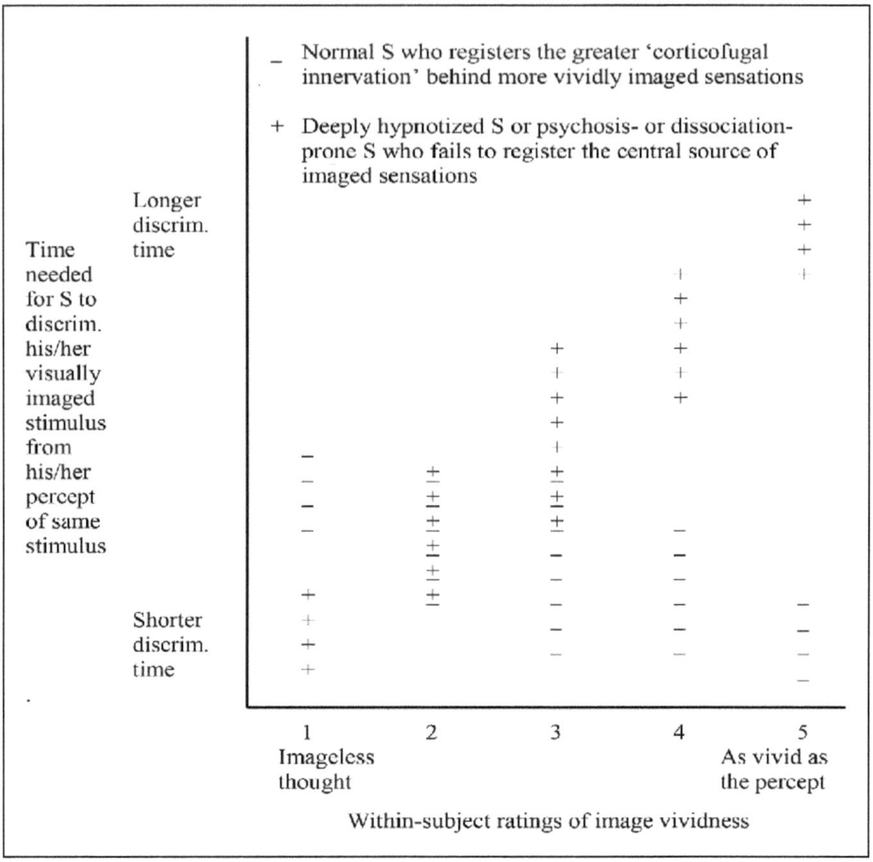

Figure 8. Two idealized 28-trial scattergrams: A normal subject's negative slope (faster image-percept discrimination times for more vivid images with greater corticofugal innervation and quicker source validation) and a hypnotized, dissociated, or psychotic subject's positive slope (slower image-percept discrimination times for more vivid images during the hypnotic, dissociative, or psychotic attenuation of self-conscious source-validation processes).

activate the source-verifying mechanism during "subliminal perceiving" merits further discussion, however, as Leibniz's (1765/1896) theoretical postulation of such perceiving and Fechner's (1860/1966) scientific study of it were building blocks in the philosophical foundations of Chapter 1.

Gottfried Leibniz's (1765/1896) notion of "petite perceptions" theoretically implied that weak stimulations of a sensory organ are normally paralleled by conscious sensations but are not necessarily accompanied by self-conscious apperception or self-consciousness that *one is "having" those sensations*. And giving scientific expression to Leibniz's notion, Gustav Fechner's (1860/1966) psychophysical equation mathematically implied that "subliminal stimuli"—stimuli exhibiting physical intensities below the "limen," the absolute threshold for self-conscious apperception—are paralleled by "negative sensations" that are not accompanied by any self-consciousness that *one is "having" those sensations*. The function of self-consciousness is not clear in Leibniz's and Fechner's formulations, but it becomes clear in Kunzendorf's source-verifying reformulation: self-consciousness that *one is "having" particular sensations* is the generic experience of either tacitly knowing that *one is perceiving those sensations* or tacitly knowing that *one is imaging those sensations*. And by implication, "petite perceptions" that are subliminally stimulated should be experienced as conscious but sourceless sensations that are readily confused with mentally imaged sensations—as the introspectionist Mary Cheves West Perky (1910) initially found to be the case. Subsequently, Kunzendorf (1984–1985) confirmed that unattended stimuli of the sort deemed "subliminal" by Corteen and Wood (1972) were memorially discriminable neither from previously imaged items nor from previously perceived items. (At the same time, control items not previously presented in the study were discriminable from the imaged items, the apperceived items, and the "subliminally" perceived items; plus the imaged items and the apperceived items were memorially discriminable from each other.) In related research, Kunzendorf and McGlinchey-Berroth (1997–1998) found that briefly presented and subsequently masked stimuli of the sort deemed "subliminal" by Jacoby and Whitehouse (1989) were discriminable from new control items when the instruction was to identify the "recently experienced (imaged or perceived)" item, but not when the instruction was to identify the "recently perceived" item. (And at the same time, self-consciously apperceived stimuli in the study were discriminable from new control items, and from imaged items, when the instruction was to identify the "recently perceived" item.) In a third study, Kunzendorf and Butler (1992) found that, during the binocular apperception of Bela Julesz's (1971) random-dot stereograms, the monocular stimulation in each eye gives rise to monocular sensations that are more likely to be misremembered as imaginal in source than either new control items or the binocular percepts are.[18]

DEFINING AND MEASURING THE SELF-CONCEPTUALIZING EXPERIENCE OF "SELF AS OBJECT"

If self-consciousness that *one is "having" (imaging or perceiving) sensory experiences* did not immediately accompany most waking experiences, then one's mind would lack a meaningful framework for conceptually distinguishing between oneself as a sensory object and other sensory objects. In order to study different primates' experience of "self as object," Gordon Gallup (1968, 1970, 1977, 1979) developed a "mirror self-recognition" paradigm for measuring the conceptualization of "self as object" in space. After preexposing different primates to mirrors, then dying one of their ears red under general anesthesia (or otherwise marking one of their body parts), Gallup discovered that only chimpanzees and orangutans seemed to recognize themselves in the mirror and tried to wipe away the red mark, indicating that chimpanzees and orangutans, like humans but unlike monkeys, possess a concept of "self as object" or a self-concept. The other warm-blooded animals that have more recently exhibited a self-concept by passing Gallup's "mark test" will be reviewed later in this chapter.

Notwithstanding the theoretical importance of differentiating self-consciousness from self-concept—"I-ness" from "me-ness" in William James' (1890) terminology, "self as subject" from "self as object" in the current terminology—many psychologists fail to distinguish between these two types of self-awareness. As Natsoulas (1989–1990) notes, psychological studies of *self-awareness* refer, sometimes, to an "apprehending state of consciousness" to which all objects of awareness "belong" and, other times, to an "apprehended state of consciousness" in which a "portion of the self [is an] object of . . . awareness" (pp. 338, 344). But notably in this regard, psychologists like Kihlstrom and Cantor (1984) mistakenly equate self-consciousness with the conscious conceptualization or representation of self, instead of recognizing that self-consciousness or "self as subject" needs to be differentiated from self-concept or "self as object."

The essential difference between self-consciousness and self-concept can be appreciated in more concrete terms, by considering Kunzendorf, McLaughlin-Beltz et al.'s (1991) two-pronged demonstration of: (a) deficient self-concepts in autistic persons; and (b) deactivated self-consciousness in hypnotized persons. In the first prong that tested for self-concept, the 36 subjects individually tested by Kunzendorf, McLaughlin-Beltz, et al. could not directly see the white line inside a 5-sided box with side-holes for inserting and moving both hands, but could see the white line indirectly in a televised mirror image. When instructed to touch the white line, 6 out of 9 autistic subjects reached toward the line on the TV (cf. Ferrari & Matthews, 1983; Spiker & Ricks, 1984)—whereas 9 out of 9 normal subjects, 8 out of 9 subjects pretending to be hypnotized, and 7 out of 9 hypnotized subjects reached toward the line inside the box. These first-prong findings thusly demonstrate that the concept of "self as object" in space (relative to other objects in space) tends to be insufficiently developed in autistic persons but tends to be normally manifested in average persons, even in the state of hypnosis. In the second prong that tested for self-consciousness, the 36 individually tested subjects moved their hands together until their fingertips touched inside the box, while ostensibly watching their hands move in real time on a mirror-imaged television screen but while actually watching a prerecorded tape of their hands moving closer together without their fingertips ever touching.

Ultimately, feeling their fingertips actually touch while watching the tape of them not touching, 7 out of 9 hypnotized subjects denied that their fingertips were touching, whereas 9 out of 9 normal subjects, 9 out of 9 subjects pretending to be hypnotized, and 8 out of 9 autistic subjects confirmed that their fingertips were touching. When asked to explain, 4 hypnotized subjects reported not being able to touch their fingertips, and 5 hypnotized subjects reported not knowing what was happening, whereas 9 out of 9 normal subjects and 9 out of 9 subjects pretending to be hypnotized reported that they must be watching a video playback of their hands, and 9 out of 9 autistic subjects reported that they didn't know what was happening. These second-prong findings demonstrate that self-consciousness that *one is perceiving tactile sensations* tends to be deactivated during the sleeplike state of hypnosis but remains active during normal wakefulness, even in autistic persons with deficient self-concepts.

DEFINING AND MEASURING THE ILLUSORY SELF-EFFICACIOUS EXPERIENCE OF "SELF AS AGENT"

Daniel Wegner's research on the illusion of "self as agent" or "the illusion of conscious will" (Wegner, 2002, 2004) indicates that "we experience conscious will when we infer that our thought causes our action" (Wegner, 2003, p. 65), which is typically "when a thought appears in consciousness just prior to an action, is consistent with the action, and appears exclusive of salient alternative causes of the action" (Wegner, 2004, p. 649). The illusory corollary that conscious will constitutes "free will" has historically been embraced by monotheists, in order to explain to themselves how evil can arise in a world created by a God who is supposedly good, according to Alexander Bain (1868). Empirical support for Bain's thesis has been obtained by Kunzendorf et al. (2008–2009)—along with empirical evidence that people who have reached Jean Piaget's (1932) stage of "moral autonomy" (after passing through a stage in which right and wrong are deemed to be God-given) do not behave as if they have "free will," but instead behave as if their moral decision-making is determined by the schemes that their minds have developed.

Just as some psychological theorists and researchers fail to differentiate "self as subject" from "self as object," so also some psychologists fail to differentiate "self as subject" from "self as agent." Notably, such failures lay the theoretical foundation for misguided conclusions concerning both the experience of lucid dreaming and the experience of self that sometimes accompanies lucid dreaming. According to Stephen LaBerge (1985), dreams become lucid when the dreamer becomes cognizant that he or she is dreaming yet continues to be asleep. The lucid dreamer's cognizance of dreaming, however, entails neither reactivation of the source-verification process on a neurological level nor self-consciousness that *one is imaging/dreaming sensations* on a subjective level—contrary to Kahan and LaBerge's (1994) contention that the lucid dreamer is self-consciously verifying the imaginal source of his or her dream imagery. Rather than being directly and incontrovertibly aware of the dream's corticofugal innervation and imaginal origins, the lucid dreamer becomes aware of the implausibility of some of the dream's contents and then *indirectly infers* that the implausible contents must be part of a dream, as documented and exemplified in research by Deirdre Barrett (1992), Kunzendorf, Treantafel, et al. (2006–2007), and LaBerge and DeGracia (2000). An illustrative example of such inferred lucidity in the absence of self-consciousness has been described by Kunzendorf (2000):

> [While] riding in the backseat of a car full of strangers, one of my students dreamed that she was being strangled by a monster, became aware that she "must be dreaming" of this monster, then nonlucidly dreamed that she had awoken and was really being strangled by the girl riding in the backseat with her. [The] bizarreness of the monster enabled her indirectly to infer that she "must be dreaming," but she was not sufficiently self-conscious to monitor the central innervation directly or to know *that she was dreaming* all the time. (p. 379)

Moreover, in Kunzendorf, Treantafel et al.'s research, 33 of the 93 lucid dreamers under study *knew* it to be *true* that "during a lucid dream, [they] have heard a real noise (e.g., an alarm clock) and have believed the noise to be part of [their] lucid dream . . . without any immediate self-awareness [of] actually perceiving the noise." In other words, lucid dreamers not only infer that their implausibly imaged sensations are being dreamed, but also infer *incorrectly* that their contemporaneously perceived sensations are being dreamed, which would not happen if their source-verification processes were activated and their centrally innervated sensations and peripherally innervated sensations were accompanied by self-consciousness that *one is imaging* and self-consciousness that *one is perceiving*, respectively.

The self-awareness that sometimes accompanies lucid dreams is, accordingly, not self-consciousness. It turns out that the experience of "self as agent," instead of the experience of "self as subject," sometimes accompanies lucid dreams. In Kunzendorf, Treantafel, et al.'s (2006–2007) study of 93 lucid dreamers, the illusory inference of "self as agent" was evident in a set of 31 lucid dreamers who reportedly "have been able to control what was happening in a dream," as well as in a subset of 24 who reportedly have experienced a dream in which "other people simply do whatever [the lucid dreamer] want[s] them or will[s] them to do [without being asked or told to do so by the lucid dreamer]." The reports of the latter 24 lucid dreamers clearly contain inferences of the sort that Wegner (2002) found necessary for the illusion of "conscious will" or of the illusion of "self as agent" to be experienced.

EVOLUTION OF SELF-AWARENESS IN MAMMALS AND BIRDS WITH PROLONGED CORTICAL DEVELOPMENT

The cross-species evidence that is pertinent to theories of "self as subject" and "self as object" does not support theories that are based on an immaterial human soul or on human language or on animal memory. Instead, this evidence indicates that self-awareness has evolved only in mammalian and avian species requiring 2 or more years to reach adulthood. Consistent with such evidence, this chapter advances the thesis that most mammals and birds who spend 2 or more years generating retinal sensations as "test images" for their developing retino-cortical rules have evolved a neural mechanism whereby visual sensations on the retina are: (a) neurally registered as "centrally innervated" or "peripherally innervated" sensations; and (b) subjectively accompanied by self-consciousness that *one is imaging or perceiving visual sensations*. Before delving into this thesis, let us briefly consider the alternatives and their shortcomings.

The neuroscientist John Eccles (1988) and other Cartesian dualists attribute self-awareness to an immaterial and immortal human soul, which is presumed not only to be *conscious of* objects outside itself, but also to be *conscious of* itself. Suggestions that self-awareness is uniquely human are not proffered only by Cartesian dualists, however: The philologist and behavioral scientist Julian Jaynes (1976) attributes self-awareness to human language, specifically to the linguistic development of first-person terminology like the analogue "I" in English. But as evidence to be detailed later in this chapter will show, self-awareness does not begin and end with the human mind (i.e., with a human soul or with human language).

The psychological scientist William James (1890) attributes self-consciousness to memory, in particular, to the "feeling of familiarity," which, when it accompanies perceptual sensations or imaginal sensations, *implies* that those sensations belong to the same self who originally experienced them. Accordingly, because memory is evident in ancient animal orders like the Blattaria order of cockroaches (Brown & Stroup, 1988; Durier & Rivault, 2001; Willner, 1978), which appeared on the evolutionary scene 400 million years ago (Kambhampati, 1995), James' memory-based theory predicts that self-awareness should arise in this order of cockroaches and in all other animal orders, except the very oldest and simplest ones.

Contrary to James' (1890) memory-based prediction and to Jaynes's (1976) language-based position, the following studies of self-recognition in mirrors suggest that self-consciousness and the self-concepts that it engenders tend to evolve in avian and mammalian species requiring 2 or more years to mature into adults with more highly developed prefrontal cortexes and more highly developed (and imaginally tested) executive routines and rules. Among birds, the Eurasian magpie, which typically requires 2 years to mature, has passed Gallup's above-described "mark test" for recognizing one's "self as object" in a mirror (Prior, Schwarz, & Güntürkün, 2008). The New Caledonian crow, requiring 4 years to mature, and the African grey parrot, requiring 6 years, have not passed Gallup's "mark test" but have passed tests similar to Kunzendorf, McLaughlin-Beltz, et al.'s (1991) above-described test for recognizing a mirrored object's spatial relationship to one's "self as object" (Medina, Taylor, Hunt, & Gray, 2011; Pepperberg, Garcia, Jackson, & Marconi, 1995). Mammals exhibiting self-recognition on Gallup's "mark test" include the human being with an average maturation period of 13 years (Broesch, Callaghan, Henrich, Murphy, & Rochat, 2011; Chapman, 1987; Gallup, Anderson, & Platek, 2003; Kärtner, Keller, Chaudhary, & Yovsi, 2012; Keller, Kärtner, Borke, Yovsi, & Kleis, 2005; Keller et al., 2004; Lewis & Ramsay, 2004; Nielsen & Dissanayake, 2004); the orangutan and the Asian elephant with an average maturation period of 12 years (Miles, 1994; Plotnik, de Waal, & Reiss, 2006; Suarez & Gallup, 1981); the bottlenose dolphin and the killer whale with an average maturation period of 10 years (Delfour & Marten, 2001; Marino, Reiss, & Gallup, 1994; Marten & Psarakos, 1994; Reiss & Marino, 2001); and the chimpanzee, the gorilla, and the bonobo with an average maturation period of 9 years (Gallup, 1970; Hyatt & Hopkins, 1994; Parker, 1994; Patterson & Cohn, 1994; Posada & Colell, 2007). In contrast, birds and mammals requiring no more than 12 months to reach sexual maturity—the Java sparrow and the dog, for example—tend to respond to their mirror image as if it is another animal (Howell & Bennett, 2011; Watanabe, 2002).

Given that the species-specific size of mature bird brains is predictive of both the duration of their maturation (Iwaniuk & Nelson, 2003) and the complexity of their concepts (Lefebvre, Reader, & Sol, 2004), it might be suggested instead that self-concepts in species requiring 2 or more years to reach maturity are attributable to greater brain size and nothing else. However, the current chapter's central thesis—that a bird or mammal who spends years refining rules by generating vivid test-images is at risk of not surviving if the bird or mammal's species has not evolved the tacit self-awareness that *one is imaging rather than perceiving*—seems more compelling from both functional and evolutionary standpoints. Evidence confirming the key assumption underlying this thesis—the assumption that the tacit experience of a "self as subject" *imaging* (or *perceiving*) *sensations* develops prior to any concept of a "self as object"—can be found in previous human-development research testing for different types of self-awareness, not in previous animal research testing only for the concept of "self as object" reflected in a mirror.

DEVELOPMENT OF SELF-AWARENESS DURING INFANCY

Research with infantile human subjects who can barely talk obviously can't employ Kunzendorf's (1980, 1985–1986a, 2000) source-verification-time paradigm that correlates each subject's image-vividness ratings with his or her image-percept discrimination times (as in Figure 8). However, as Wyman, Rakoczy, and Tomasello (2009) note, infantile "pretence presupposes some implicit pretend-reality distinction (otherwise pretending children would be considered delusional) and this implicit understanding is evident in the ability of 2-year-olds to engage in joint inferential pretence" with objects (p. 388).[19] Moreover, three longitudinal studies of human infants have confirmed that the shift from self-oriented play to source-verified play with objects of pretense develops prior to the shift from mirror-image "mark test" failure to mirror-image self-recognition. In studying a group of 10 infants, Michael Chapman (1987) found that the shift away from self-oriented play occurred before 18 months of age and the shift away from "mark test" failures occurred after 18 months; but in another group of 9 infants, he found that both shifts occurred after 18 months of age. In a second study involving 77 infants, Nielsen and Dissanayake (2004) found that most of the shift to pretend play with objects occurred before 18 months of age, whereas much of the shift to self-recognition in a mirror occurred after 18 months. In a third study of 66 infants, Lewis and Ramsay (2004) found that the shift to pretend play with objects occurred before 18 months of age, whereas the shift to self-recognition in a mirror occurred after 18 months. And like Wyman et al. (2009), Lewis and Ramsay (2004) noted the implicit source-verifying ability underlying pretend play:

> The child feeding a doll imaginary food or the child drinking an imaginary liquid from a cup must know that what he or she is doing is not real. If children did not know that their actions on objects were not real, their play would not be pretense, but a hallucination. (p. 1821)

The cross-cultural research literature similarly shows that pretend play accompanied by self-consciousness that *one is imaging objects of play* develops before the concept of "self as object" in a mirror. Thus, self-consciousness that *one is pretending* is evident in all African, Chinese, Euro-American, and Indian toddlers (Bloch & Adler, 1994; Haight, Wang, Fung, Williams, & Mintz, 1999; Roopnarine, Hossain, Gill, & Brophy, 1994). In contrast, the concept of "self as object" in a mirror is evident in a low percentage of African toddlers, a moderate to high percentage of Euro-American toddlers, and a low to moderate percentage of Indian toddlers (Broesch et al., 2011; Kärtner et al., 2012; Keller et al., 2004, 2005).

Self-consciousness that *one is pretending* turns out to be one of the earliest executive functions to develop in human prefrontal cortex (De Luca & Leventer, 2008; German, Niehaus, Roarty, Giesbrecht, & Miller, 2004; Leslie, 1987). And consistent with the thesis of this chapter, the development of all other prefrontal executive functions comes to completion near the end of adolescence (De Luca & Leventer, 2008), when the frequency and the vividness of all mental imagery, including "test imagery," begin to decline (Giambra, 2000).

SOME HUMANS' GENETIC PROPENSITY FOR DEACTIVATING SELF-CONSCIOUS SOURCE VERIFICATION

As noted in Chapter 1 as well as in this chapter, all adult human beings deactivate the self-conscious source-verification system during sleep and dreaming. However, a tendency to deactivate the self-conscious verification of wakefully imaged or wakefully perceived stressors has evolved in some people, whereas a tendency to remain self-conscious during all wakeful experiences has evolved in others.

Psychotic Hallucinating: Deactivating the Self-Conscious Source Verification of Wakefully Imagined Stressors

Based on their phenomenological studies with schizophrenic patients, Sass and Parnas (2003) argue that

> although the major symptoms and signs of schizophrenia are heterogeneous in many respects, they can nevertheless be understood in a fairly unified way [as] a self-disorder or, more specifically . . . a diminishment of . . . the implicit sense of existing as a vital and self-possessed subject of awareness . . . in a way that involves no distinction between a subject and an object. (p. 428)

Schizophrenia implies no distinction between a subjectively generated image (a psychotic hallucination) and an objectively stimulated percept in other words. Consistent with this phenomenological understanding of psychosis, studies of self-conscious source verification show that diminished self-consciousness of the imaginal origins of self-generated sensations and the perceptual origins of object-elicited sensations is associated with psychosis-proneness in the general population (Kunzendorf, 2000; Kunzendorf, Moran, et al., 1995–1996) and with hallucination-severity in the schizophrenic population (Aleman, Böcker, Hijman, de Haan, & Kahn, 2003; Böcker, Hijman, Kahn, & de Haan, 2000; Mintz & Alpert, 1972). And consistent with Figure 8's paradigmatic illustration that hallucinating entails less source verification, but not necessarily more vivid imaging, additional studies indicate that schizophrenics' images are no more vivid than other people's images (Brett & Starker, 1977; Chandiramani & Varma, 1987; Starker, 1979; Starker & Jolin, 1983–1984). In paranoid schizophrenia, diminished self-conscious image-verification should serve to multiply the impact of any vivid emotion-provoking image—given Kunzendorf, Francis, et al.'s (1996–1997) finding that the fight/flight-evoking image of being in a hijacked airplane raises systolic blood pressure 18 mmHg in people exhibiting both more vivid imagery and less proficient source verification, but does not raise it significantly in anyone else. In thought-disordered schizophrenia, diminished self-consciousness should serve not only to attenuate the verification of whether sensations represent self-generated images or object-elicited percepts, but also to attenuate the verification of whether successively uttered words reflect self-intended associations or object-elicited associations (Cohen & Camhi, 1967; Cohen, Nachmani, & Rosenberg, 1974; Kantorowitz & Cohen, 1977) as well as the verification of whether individual words in short-term memory represent utterances or thoughts (Nienow & Docherty, 2004). Notably, in research into schizophrenics' attenuated ability to verify whether words were self-generated or not, Costafreda, Brébion, Allen, McGuire, and Fu (2008) and Morrison and Haddock (1997) discovered that schizophrenic hallucinators' source-verification ability was especially diminished when the words had emotional connotations.

Psychotic features are prevalent not only in 61%–94% of patients under treatment for schizophrenia (Ndetei & Singh, 1983; Sedman, 1966; Zarroug, 1975), but also in 80% of patients under treatment for bipolar depression (McElroy, Strakowski, West, Keck, & McConville, 1997) and 25% of patients under treatment for major depression (Coryell, Pfohl, & Zimmerman, 1984). Moreover, studies of identical-twin pairings with one schizophrenic twin and one bipolar twin suggest that schizophrenic psychosis and depressive psychosis share some genetic underpinnings (Cardno, Rijsdijk, Sham, Murray, & McGuffin, 2002; McGuffin, Reveley, & Holland, 1982). But at the same time, studies of "depressive realism" suggest that people who suffer from depression *without psychosis* are more in touch with reality than nondepressed people (Alloy & Abramson, 1979, 1988; Kunzendorf & McLaughlin, 1988–1989; Nelson & Craighead, 1977; Powell & Hemsley, 1984; Roth & Ingram, 1985; Sackeim, 1983; Zung & Gianturco, 1971). Consistent with both of these suggestions, Kunzendorf, Moran, et al.'s (1995–1996) study found that depressed college students whose interpretations of reality were imbued with "negative meaning" and with negative distortion exhibited source-verification deficits (i.e., exhibited positive slopes on Figure 8's source-verification-time exercise), whereas depressed students whose interpretations of reality were imbued with "no meaning" and with existential authenticity exhibited negative slopes on Figure's 8's source-verification-time exercise.

The latter studies, when considered in light of the author's experience treating a schizo-affective hallucinator, raise the possibility that persons with the genetic propensity to attenuate the source-verification process for negative imagery can defend themselves in this manner, whereas persons without such a genetic propensity must remain self-consciously "in touch" with any negative imagery and any depressing self-knowledge thereby engendered. The schizo-affective hallucinator in question, whom I treated for panic attacks during my clinical externship in the Behavioral Medicine Program at Cambridge Hospital, reported that she frequently saw her deceased brother's ghost tying a noose and holding it out for her to hang herself. On account of her lack of self-consciousness that *she was imaging her brother and the noose,* she was able to defend herself against the depressing self-knowledge: (a) that the source of the hallucinatory image of the noose was in her own mind; and (b) that her mind harbored suicidal impulses. But even with her lack of self-conscious source verification, she had the option of *inferring* either that her visual sensations of her brother were the product of her own imagination, given their faintness, or that her visual sensations were the ghost of her brother, given that a "ghost or wraith need not be fully lifelike [or vivid] to be seen 'out there' as something present in space" (Hilgard, 1981, p. 14). By opting for the latter inference—the psychotic inference—she defended herself against inferential self-knowledge that the urge to commit suicide originated within herself. And by implication, if she had not had the genetic propensity to attenuate the self-conscious source-verification system during wakefulness, then her only option would have been to experience directly the disturbing and depressing self-awareness that *her brother's noose was a self-generated image*, an image that gave visual expression to the suicidal impulses within her.[20]

Dissociating: Deactivating the Self-Conscious Source Verification of Wakefully Perceived Stressors

Whereas an attenuated source-verification process enables the hallucination-prone person to avoid awareness of the self-generation of disturbing images and to psychotically attribute perceptual origins to such images, an attenuated source-verification process enables the dissociation-prone person to avoid awareness of the reality of disturbing percepts and to dissociatively attribute imaginal origins to such percepts (Kunzendorf, 2000, 2006). Thus, as Kunzendorf (2006, 2010) and Lynn, Lilienfeld, Merckelbach, Giesbrecht, and van der Kloet (2012) summarily note, and as Kunzendorf (1989–1990) and Kunzendorf and Moran (1993–1994) empirically demonstrate, dissociation from a threatening percept does not yield reversible amnesia on account of the perceptual experience being actively repressed, but instead yields irreversible "source amnesia" on account of the percept having been encoded as "not real" during deactivated source verification. And due to such "source amnesia," the threatening percept can be reexperienced only as a recollection that is "not real"—that is, as an "unbidden image," the origins of which can be inferred to be imaginary or "subconscious" or sourceless.

The present position—that dissociative disorders share psychotic disorders' underlying deficiency in self-conscious source verification—is supported by one set of studies associating dissociative psychopathology with psychotic phenomena, including image-verification deficits, and by another set of studies associating psychotic psychopathology with dissociative phenomena, including percept-verification deficits. In one of two studies from the latter set, Kilcommons and Morrison (2005) administered the Positive and Negative Syndrome Scale (the PANSS; Kay, Fiszbein, & Opler, 1987) and the Dissociative Experiences Scale (the DES; Bernstein & Putnam, 1986) to 16 psychiatric patients with a diagnosis of schizophrenia, plus 16 patients with other psychiatric diagnoses, and they discovered that the PANSS hallucinations total score was significantly correlated with both the DES depersonalization factor score ($r = .59$) and the DES amnesic dissociation factor score ($r = .52$). In the other study, Perona-Garcelán et al. (2012) administered the Cambridge Depersonalization Scale (the CDS; Sierra & Berrios, 2000) to 27 schizophrenic hallucinators, plus 22 patients with other psychiatric diagnoses, and they obtained significantly higher CDS scores from the schizophrenic hallucinators.

The set of studies associating dissociative psychopathology with psychotic phenomena, on the other hand, includes investigations of people exhibiting a broad range of dissociative disorders and dissociative phenomena. Three investigations into the most severe dissociative phenomenon—Multiple Personality Disorder (MPD), now called Dissociative Identity Disorder (DID)[21]—uncovered auditory hallucinating in 47% of the 30 MPD patients studied by Richard Kluft (1987), 81% of the 102 MPD patients studied by Ross et al. (1990), and 72% of the 236 MPD patients studied by Ross, Norton, and Wozney (1989). And in an investigation into the full spectrum of dissociative phenomena, Allen, Coyne, and Console (1997) administered the DES and the Millon Clinical Multiaxial Inventory (the MCMI; Millon, 1994) to 226 psychiatric patients with trauma-related disorders, and they discovered that the DES total score was significantly correlated with the MCMI psychotic "thought disorder" scale ($r = .69$) and the MCMI schizotypal personality scale ($r = .57$). Furthermore, six investigations into the dissociative experiences of college students found that higher DES scores are statistically associated with poorer source verification (Dehon, Bastin, & Larøi, 2008; Heaps & Nash, 1999; Hyman & Billings, 1998; Kunzendorf & Karpen, 1996–1997; Wilkinson & Hyman, 1998; Winograd, Peluso, & Glover, 1998). Indeed, Kunzendorf and Karpen's (1996–1997) investigation found that higher DES scores are associated with positive slopes on Figure 8's source-verification exercise, just as Kunzendorf, Moran, et al.'s (1995–1996) study found that higher psychoticism scores are associated with positive slopes on Figure 8's source-verification-time exercise—where positive slopes indicate that perceived sensations are no longer discriminated more quickly from more vividly imaged sensations, presumably because quicker self-conscious verification of the greater centrifugal innervation underlying more vividly imaged sensations is defunct in the psychotic state of mind and the dissociated state of mind.

Finally, just as the author's previously described experience of treating a schizo-affective hallucinator raises the possibility that persons with the inherited ability to deactivate the self-conscious source-verification system can use such an ability to convince themselves that undesirable mental images are not self-generated, an empirical study by Kunzendorf, Hulihan, Simpson, Pritykina, and Williams (1997–1998) raises the possibility that people with this inherited ability can also use it to convince themselves that undesired perceptual experiences are not real. Kunzendorf et al. (1997–1998) studied psychiatric patients who were deemed by their therapists to have definitely suffered physical or sexual abuse—42 patients with dissociation-related diagnoses, 30 patients with nonpsychotic depression-related diagnoses, and 34 patients with anxiety-related diagnoses. All patients were administered Tellegen and Atkinson's (1974) "absorption" scale measuring the trait of "openness to absorbing and self-altering experiences" (p. 268), a trait with 50% heritability (Tellegen et al., 1988). Half of the patients whose absorption scores were above the median manifested dissociation-related diagnoses in response to abuse, whereas three quarters of the patients whose absorption scores were below the median manifested depression-related or anxiety-related diagnoses in response to abuse. In other words, the patients with an inherited propensity for absorption in fantasy and for openness to self-altering experiences tended to be patients who deactivated self-conscious source verification during their abuse and who subsequently experienced source amnesia for their abuse, "unbidden images" of their abuse, and other signs and symptoms that dissociated them from the reality of their abuse. In contrast, the patients without such an inherited propensity tended to be patients whose perceptions of abuse were self-consciously verified and whose memories of abuse were depressingly real.

A Genetic Propensity to Deactivate the Source-Verification Process in Psychosis and Dissociation

The current suggestion that the wakeful deactivation of the self-conscious source-verification system underlies both psychotic hallucinating and dissociative source amnesia is anticipated by long-standing arguments for a "unitary concept of mental illness" (Menninger, Ellenberger, Pruyser, & Mayman, 1958, p. 4), and it anticipates 21st century research into the common genetic underpinnings of psychotic and dissociative psychopathology. In the former regard, one of the strongest and most recent champions of the unitary concept, Andrew Moskowitz, finds that "voices heard by persons diagnosed schizophrenic appear to be indistinguishable, on the basis of their experienced characteristics, from voices heard by persons with dissociative disorders" (Moskowitz & Corstens, 2007, pp. 35–36). Accordingly, as former NIMH director Steven Hyman observes, "Many people who get one diagnosis get five diagnoses, but they don't have five diseases—they have one underlying condition" (Belluck & Carey, 2013, p. A15). And as current NIMH director Thomas Insel further observes, "People think that everything has to match [official diagnostic] criteria, but . . . Biology never read that book" (Belluck & Carey, 2013, p. A12).

In the latter regard, recent genetic studies indicate that both psychotic psychopathology and dissociative psychopathology are statistically associated with the Val/Val genotype of the COMT (catechol-O-methyltransferase) gene. In psychosis-related studies, the Val/Val genotype has been found in 25% of schizophrenic patients ($n = 40$; Abdolmaleky et al., 2006) to 61% of schizophrenic patients ($n = 59$; Goghari & Sponheim, 2008), and in 30% of bipolar patients with psychotic histories ($n = 230$; Benedetti et al., 2010; DeRosse, Malhotra, & Lencz, 2012). The Val/Val genotype was found in only 10% of nonpsychiatric medical patients in a control group ($n = 40$; Abdolmaleky et al., 2006). And for 37 mood-disordered patients exhibiting the COMT Val/Val genotype (but not for 141 patients exhibiting either the COMT Met/Met genotype or the COMT Val/Met genotype), higher DES dissociativity scores were statistically associated with greater amounts of reported abuse on Bernstein et al.'s (2003) Childhood Trauma Questionnaire (Savitz et al., 2008). Given such genetic research findings, DeRosse et al. (2012) conclude that genotypes like the Val/Val genotype are associated with psychotic features across diagnostic categories, not with any particular psychiatric diagnosis. And to the extent the Val/Val genotype is associated with not only with psychotic inferences regarding the source of discomforting fantasies, but also with dissociative inferences regarding the source of discomforting realities, the above findings do seem to point toward a "unitary concept of mental illness" based on the inherited ability to deactivate the self-conscious source-verification system during wakeful discomfort.

If the concluding thesis of this chapter is correct, then human self-consciousness has been evolving in two diverging directions. On one hand, the ability to defend against discomforting images and discomforting percepts by deactivating the self-conscious source-verification system during wakefulness seems to have been evolving in a subpopulation of humans with the COMT Val/Val genotype. Abdolmaleky et al.'s (2006) documentation of this genotype not only in 25% of their schizophrenic subjects but also in 10% of their normal control subjects suggests that this wakeful ability serves as a latent defense mechanism, which remains dormant unless the need to make psychotic inferences that discomforting images are perceptual in origin (or dissociative inferences that discomforting percepts are imaginal in origin) arises in someone with the Val/Val genotype. On the other hand, the inability to deactivate the self-conscious source-verification system during wakefulness seems to have been evolving in humans who exhibit neither the Val/Val genotype nor any other genotype associated with psychotic hallucinating and dissociative amnesia.

This apparent divergence in the evolution of human self-consciousness has important implications for the survival of our species, when considered in the light of research suggesting that self-consciousness of the reality of others may serve to prevent wakefully self-conscious humans from doing actual harm to others. In this regard, studies by Arseneault, Moffitt, Caspi, Taylor, and Silva (2000) and by Brennan, Mednick, and Hodgins (2000) suggest that psychotic people's propensity to deactivate the self-awareness that *discomforting fantasies are self-generated images* can serve also to deactivate self-consciousness that *people to whom one might like to respond with violence are real people.* In a similar vein, research reviewed by Eugene Bliss (1986) and by Andrew Moskowitz (2004) suggests that dissociatively disordered people's propensity to deactivate self-consciousness that *one is really being abused* can serve to deactivate self-consciousness that *one is really abusing others.* But still, individuals with the wakeful propensity to deactivate the self-conscious source-verification system retain the ability to *infer* that their vivid sensations of other people are sensory experiences of real people—an ability that needs to be cultivated not only by reality-focalizing psychotherapy but also by reality-focusing political rhetoric and reality accommodating religious technology, lest someone with an inherited propensity to deactivate self-consciousness and with an acquired weapon of mass destruction do widespread harm to real people of every genotype.

EPILOGUE: CONSCIOUSNESS OF THE SELF AND THE DEATH OF SELF

According to this fourth and final chapter, consciousness of "self as subject" is the subjective aspect of neurally verifying that *one is imaging sensations* (or *perceiving them*), is a survival-promoting aspect of certain warm-blooded animals who spend 2 or more years constructing "test images" from their developing cortical rules, and is a prerequisite for self-concepts such as the "self as object" recognized in mirror-images. The existential anthropologist Ernest Becker (1973) has noted that self-consciousness is also a prerequisite for conceptualizing both the death of "self as bodily object" and the death of "self as subject":

> What does it mean to be a *self-conscious animal?* . . . It means to know that one is food for worms. This is the terror: to have emerged from nothing, to have . . . consciousness of self, deep inner feelings, an excruciating inner yearning for life and self-expression—and with all this yet to die. (p. 87)

It is all too frequently assumed that only a human being can self-consciously imagine the death of oneself. But if the hypotheses put forth in this chapter are correct, then a mammal or bird who requires 2 or more years to reach sexual and cognitive maturity might also be capable of self-consciously imagining the death of oneself. All such an animal needs to do is self-consciously imagine being consumed by a lion or by worms or by the earth beneath one's feet. After asking "What mental image is present when I think of the death of myself?" the phenomenologist Peter Koestenbaum (1964–1965) answered, "Honest analysis will disclose that there is then no image of the world left [just] an encounter with nothingness" (pp. 142–143). So we should not be surprised that, when asked "What is death?" with sign language, the gorilla Koko has reportedly signed back that death is "a warm hole" (http://aboutfacts.net/MotherEarth35.htm). Nor should we be surprised that, when observed in the wild, some chimpanzees, some elephants, and some magpies have purposively buried their dead (Bradshaw, 2004; Pierce, 2012; R. K. Siegel, 1980), for more than they fear death itself, self-conscious organisms fear a meaningless or purposeless death (Becker, 1975; Kunzendorf, Leszkiewicz, et al., 2006–2007). The problem of finding meaning in the context of one's mortality is a problem that has arisen out of the evolution of self-consciousness, to be sure, but it is a problem that is beyond the scope of this book and is addressed in a separate line of research by this author (Kunzendorf, 1985–1986b, 2007a; Kunzendorf & Buker, 2007–2008; Kunzendorf, DeJesus, Chicos, & Avalos, 2000–2001; Kunzendorf, Doherty, Visconti, Giacalone, & Vangapalli, 2015–2016; Kunzendorf, Leszkiewicz, Hamill, McAleer, Geoffroy, Ciampaglia, Pereira, Brito, 2006–2007; Kunzendorf & McLaughlin, 1988–1989).

APPENDIX A

Introspective Exercise Demonstrating Binocular Illusion of Fused Sensations

When both eyes are simultaneously focused on a faraway set of objects at different distances, we are unaware of the two eyes' separate visual sensations for two reasons: because such a faraway set of objects produces nearly identical sensations on the two eyes' retinas and because the brain does not not register whether particular sensations are present in one eye or both eyes (Kunzendorf et al., 1988). But when both eyes are simultaneously focused on a closeby set of objects at different distances, we often experience binocularly disparate sensations and sometimes experience an illusion of binocularly fused sensations.

The following exercise for demonstrating the binocular illusion of fused sensations was developed by Kunzendorf (2007b). For purposes of this demonstration, one needs to sit down with one's hands on one's knees and to point one's index fingers toward each other with one's fingertips touching, while looking through the fingers to the floor until one sees the binocular disparity depicted in Figure 9(a). As soon as one sees this disparity, one should keep staring cross-eyed through one's touching fingertips while slowly rotating one's fingers until they form a right angle pointing away from one's body. At this point, by selectively focusing attention on the two eyes' sensations, one can binocularly abstract either the diamond depicted in Figure 9(c) or the heart depicted in Figure 9(d). If one instead focuses one's attention on the left eye's sensations, one's binocular abstraction will resemble Figure 9(e); or if one focuses one's attention on the right eye's sensations, one's binocular abstraction will resemble Figure 9(f); and if one looks at one's fingers instead of through them, one's binocular abstraction will resemble Figure 9(b). So long as one continues to stare through one's fingers to the floor, both eyes' sensations can be experienced, but the particular sensations belonging to each eye cannot be cortically computed or tacitly known (Kunzendorf et al., 1988; Ono & Barbeito, 1985); at the same time, either a binocularly structured diamond or a binocularly structured heart can be

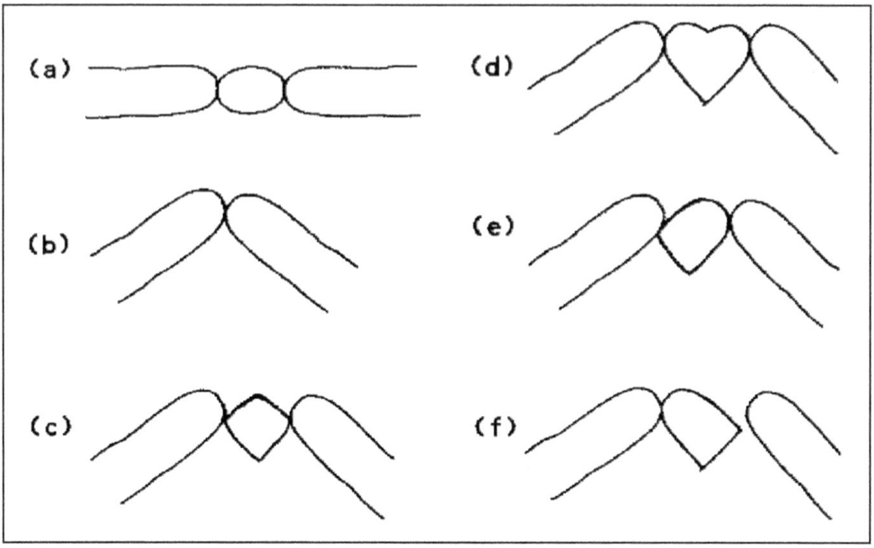

Figure 9. Percepts of fingertips: (a) binocular percept of fingertips pointing straight at each other and touching a fleshy ellipsoid; (b) monocular percept of fingertips touching perpendicular to each other; (c) binocular percept of fingertips oriented perpendicularly and separated by a fleshy diamond; (d) binocular percept of fingertips oriented perpendicularly and separated by a fleshy heart; (e) binocular percept of 1.5 perpendicular fingertips from left eye and 1 fingertip from right eye; (f) binocular percept of 1.5 fingertips from right eye and 1 fingertip from left eye. Adapted from "Is Binocular Fusion of 'Cortical Yellow' an Illusion, Contingent Upon Abstraction of Coherent Sensory Information From the Two Eyes?" by R. G. Kunzendorf (2007b). Reproduced with permission.

cortically abstracted from the two eyes' sensations and can be tacitly experienced as an inferred shape in relation to both eyes' sensations.

This demonstration not only supports Sir Charles Sherrington's (1911) position—that binocular fusion leads to a unified interpretation of both eyes' sensations, not to a unified cortical array of sensations—but also supports Hermann von Helmholtz's (1910/1962) position:

> I am led to conclude that any anatomical hypothesis which assumes that the sensations in the two eyes are completely fused with each other . . . is inadmissible and incompatible with the facts. . . . The form of the union of the impressions in the visual fields of the two eyes is the apperception of material things. Where this does not succeed on account of the nature of the two images, the attention will waver, as shown by the rivalry between the two visual globes, unless the attention is riveted by sharply defined outlines in one of the fields. (pp. 539–541)

APPENDIX B

On the Role of Pain in Basic Negative Emotions

The three basic negative emotions—anger, fear, and sadness—can certainly be painful. The empirically interesting and theoretically important possibility is that these three subjective qualities and their neural underpinnings may have evolved from the three basic pain receptors—the heat nociceptor, the chemical nociceptor, and the pressure nociceptor, respectively.

In describing anger, the epic poet Homer (c. 800 BCE/2006) wrote, "My blood boils when I think it all over and remember how [he] treated me with contumely as though I were some vile tramp" (p. 75). Consistent with Homer's poetic description of blood-boiling or heat-generating anger, the bodily sensation that 3,364 research subjects from 39 countries differentially associated with anger was "feeling hot" (Breugelmans et al., 2005; Scherer & Wallbott, 1994). Thus, it seems plausible that the sympathetic nervous system's subjective aspect of painful *heated anger* and its parallel physical aspect of *fighting off* the pain's stimulant may have evolved from heat nociception.

In describing fear, the epic poet John Milton (1674/1962) wrote, "My inbred enemy . . . tore through my entrails . . . with fear and pain" (p. 52). Consistent with Milton's description of gut-wrenching fear, the bodily complaints that 2,237 research subjects from two disparate cultures differentially associated with fear were pain in the stomach, indigestion, and diarrhea (Beirens & Fontaine, 2010). Thus, it seems plausible that the sympathetic nervous system's subjective aspect of painful *gut-wrenching fear* and its parallel physical aspect of *fleeing* or otherwise avoiding the pain's stimulant may have evolved from chemical nociception.

And in describing sadness, the poet Robert Frost wrote, "A poem begins with a lump in the throat: a homesickness or a love-sickness" (Untermeyer, 1951, p. 240). Confirming Frost's association of sadness with a pressure or lump in the throat, the bodily sensation which 3,364 research subjects from 39 countries differentially associated with sadness was a lump in the throat (Breugelmans et al., 1994). Thus, it also seems plausible that the reptilian nervous system's subjective aspect of painful *pressure-in-the-throat sadness* and its parallel physical aspect of *freezing* (not moving) upon contact with the pain's stimulant may have evolved from pressure nociception.

In addressing the evolutionary function of positive affect, Robert Levenson (1994) suggested "that positive emotions might be associated with a state of physiological quiescence, and that their primary function might be to '*undo*' the autonomic activation produced by negative emotions" (p. 256). Let us briefly consider the particular positive emotions that seem to be associated with the resolution or "undoing" of each of the three basic negative emotions.

When anger is resolved, one of two positive feelings may be implicated. On one hand, if *anger* and its behavioral disposition to *fight* a threat are resolved through conquest, then a feeling of *triumph* may follow—a feeling that Carroll Izard (1978) equates with intense *happiness*. (Of course, as Izard notes, this triumphant form of happiness may also follow conquests unrelated to anger: scientific conquests, for instance.) On the other hand, if *anger* and the disposition to *fight* a threat are positively resolved without actual fighting and without further threat, then a feeling of *contentment* may follow. So feelings of triumph and contentment appear to be two variations of happiness, both of which represent positive resolutions of negative anger.

When *fear* and its behavioral disposition to *flee* a threat are positively resolved, a feeling of relief may follow. And when *sadness* and its behavioral disposition to *freeze* in response to real or imagined loss are resolved, *interest* in the world is restored. In the latter regard, Kunzendorf et al.'s (2000–2001) research on emotional responses to music has demonstrated that interest does indeed serve to "undo" sadness.

Finally, it is noteworthy that vividly imaging either an emotion or its environmental stimulant tends to trigger the emotion's autonomic concomitants (McMahon, 1973, 1974, 1976). Accordingly, as demonstrated in research reviewed by Barber (1984), Sheikh and Kunzendorf (1984), and Sheikh, Kunzendorf, Sheikh, and Baer (2003), vivid imaging can induce changes in heart rate, blood pressure, blood flow, body chemistry, and immune responding.

Endnotes

1. Although it is often claimed that the "intelligent design" movement is not religious, Michael Powell (2005) quotes the movement's founder, Phillip Johnson, as saying that "if the pure Darwinist account was accurate and life is all about an undirected material process, then Christian metaphysics and religious belief are fantasy" (p. 12). Ironically, Johnson's understanding of Christian metaphysics seems not to be informed by the many Biblical passages promising Christians material salvation through bodily resurrection after death. Neither the undirected evolution of conscious brains nor the death of nerve cells and their conscious qualities is at odds with the Christian doctrine of the resurrection of the body, as John J. C. Smart (1967) makes clear in his encyclopedic treatise on science and religion.
2. Cognitive scientist Steven Kosslyn's (1994) theoretical reduction of the subjectively experienced image to an objectively represented analogue has led to a three-decade-long debate with cognitive scientist Zenon Pylyshyn (1973, 1981, 2003) over whether visual thoughts are imagistic analogues or imageless propositions—a debate that Kunzendorf et al. (2013-2014) have reframed into an issue of individual differences between imageless heterarchical thinkers and imageless hierarchical thinkers. But on a purely theoretical level, Kosslyn's reductionist approach has no bearing on the debate between psychological scientists over whether visually imaged sensations are contained in all thoughts or are constructed from imageless thoughts. Indeed, given Kosslyn's (1994) assertion that the "term 'image' [should] refer to the internal representation that is used in information processing, not the experience itself" (p. 3), a psychological scientist could conclude either that Kosslyn is studying the physical substrates paralleling visually imaged sensations or that he is studying the physical substrates of the imageless thoughts from which visually imaged sensations are sometimes constructed, sometimes not.
3. Color constancies have to be calculated from juxtaposed sensations of color. For example, as I look down at my brown shoes on the green carpet, the desktop is casting a shadow over my left foot. Consequently, the brownish sensations composing my left shoe are darker than the brownish sensation composing my right shoe, and the greenish sensations composing carpet on the left are darker than the greenish sensations composing carpet on the right. But at the same time, my nervous system calculates that the brightness ratio of dark-brown-to-dark-green on the left is equivalent to the brightness ratio of light-brown-to-light-green on the right, and my sensations are

paralleled by the imageless implication that I am wearing two shoes of constant brownness and need not change either one of them.

4. During normal dreaming and during lucid dreaming, the sleeping brain fails to register and verify the central innervation of dreamed sensations, and the sleeping mind fails to be self-conscious that *one is imaging rather than perceiving*. But during lucid dreaming, the sleeping person comes to believe that he or she is dreaming by using dream content (e.g., bizarre sensations) to infer that he or she is dreaming all the sensory contents not by self-consciously verifying whether the source of the dreamed sensations is imaginal or perceptual. Thus, in research by Kunzendorf, Treantafel et al. (2006–2007), 35% of the 93 lucid dreamers *knew* it to be *true* that "during a lucid dream, [they] have heard a real noise (an alarm clock, e.g.) and have believed the noise to be part of [their] lucid dream . . . without any immediate self-awareness [of] actually perceiving the noise."
5. Although Fechner's (1860/1966) logarithmic equation continues to relate sensory magnitude to physical intensity within certain boundary conditions, it has been superseded by S. S. Stevens' (1961) power law.
6. Corals, anemones, and most jellyfish reproduce *asexually* by breaking off or splitting, or *sexually* by depositing eggs in water and spraying them with sperm (Animal Life Resource, 2012a, 2012b). According to Christine Hoekenga (2012) from the Smithsonian Institution's Museum of Natural History, one species of jellyfish—*Carybdea sivickisi*, a box jelly—exhibits a courtship ritual or mating dance. In the Anthropoda phylum that subsequently evolved, however, 91 of the 343 genera of water mites studied by Heather Proctor (1991) evolved copulation, and none of the 343 genera showed signs of reversing to noncopulative spawning—consistent with the evolutionary axiom that sexual pleasure promotes copulation and thereby promotes survival of the species and genus.
7. Andrew Parker (2003) suggests that ocelli's pigment patches "may have evolved rather as a light barrier—to absorb light and so shield the underlying sensory cells that detect other stimuli" (p. 189).
8. Avian eyes normally contain four different types of cones with lightwave-responsiveness peaking around 375–400 nm (violet), 450–470 nm (blue), 540 nm (green-yellow), and 600 nm (yellow-orange) (Osorio & Vorobyev, 2008; Rojas, McNeil, Cabana, & Lachapelle, 1999a, 1999b), and human eyes normally contain three types of cones with responsiveness peaking around 435 nm (blue-violet), 530 nm (green), and 560 nm (yellow-green) (Merbs & Nathans, 1992a, 1992b; Schnapf, Kraft, & Baylor, 1987). However, some human females possess mutated eyes containing four types of cones with lightwave-responsiveness peaking around 435 nm (blue-violet), 530 nm (green), 545 nm (green-yellow), and 560 nm (yellow-green); plus half of the male offspring of such females possess mutated eyes containing three red/green color-blind cones with responsiveness peaking either around 435 nm (blue-violet), 530 nm (green), and 545 nm (green-yellow) or around 435 nm (blue-violet), 545 nm (green-yellow), and560 nm (yellow-green) (Jordan et al., 2010).
9. The only time the introspective experience of a color changes along with its surrounding context is when the surround alters the retinal excitation itself, as in lateral inhibition.
10. The current findings suggest that just as sensations of yellow are not cortically constructed from cone-cell signals stimulated by both red and green wavelengths, so

also sensations of white are not cortically constructed from cone-cell signals stimulated by the spectrum of wavelengths composing white light. Consistent with this suggestion regarding sensations of white, Peachey, Alexander, Fishman, and Derlacki (1989) employed a rod-saturating background for flash electroretinograms (ERGs) and unexpectedly found that the b-wave of photopic (cone-cell) ERGs does not increase in amplitude as white flashes get more and more intense. The latter finding can easily be explained, however, if white sensations are posited to be the subjective aspects of rod cells rather than the subjective aspects of cortical white-sensing neurons that can be innervated either by rod-cell signals or by a cross-spectrum mixture of cone-cell signals.

11. The main reason for generating visually imaged sensations from a sensationless schema such as the set of rules governing depth and size constancy is to test newly hypothesized and newly refined rules in the schema, without bumping one's head against reality. This hypothesis-testing function of mental images was introduced in Chapter 1 and will be developed further in Chapter 3.
12. The fact that sensations sometimes seem to be disrupted by cortical lesions is often interpreted as demonstrating that sensations are subjective qualities of cortical neurons. Of course, what is disrupted may be tacit cortical inferences in relation to sensations rather than sensations per se (as seems to be the case in "blindsight," which is discussed in Endnote 17). But no matter whether sensations or sensationless inferences are disrupted by cortical lesions, research by Derek Denny-Brown (1966), S. Murray Sherman (1974), and James Sprague (1966) shows that subsequent lesions sometimes counter the effects of initial lesions and sometimes restore the sensations or inferences that were initially disrupted. Interpretations of the disruptive effects of cortical lesions should accordingly remain open to the possibility that subsequent lesions might disrupt those disruptive effects.
13. Whereas Wolter (1965a, 1991) reportedly observed tens of thousands of centrifugal fibers per human retina, Repérant and Gallego (1976) reportedly observed fewer than 10 centrifugal fibers per human retina. Although this huge discrepancy is not readily reconciled, it might possibly be integrated into this chapter's thesis that huge individual differences in the vividness of human beings' visual imaging at the retinal level are indications: (a) that children and artists centrifugally construct vivid retinal images from imageless cortical rules in order to test and refine their developing rules; and (b) that most adults stop using their corticofugal pathways to construct vivid retinal images (and let their retinopetal pathways atrophy) as soon as their cortical rules are sufficient to navigate visually and to survive. Although this integrative hypothesis regarding differences in centrifugal fiber counts remains to be tested, it is noteworthy that Wolter observed centrifugal-fiber regeneration in his 1960 study of the enucleated eye from a 4-year-old boy but not in his 1979 study of the enucleated eye from a 56-year-old man.
14. Wolter and Knoblich (1965) discovered that, whereas afferent fibers from the retina atrophy quite rapidly following total blindness, centrifugal fibers can survive as long as 50 years after the onset of total blindness. By implication, it may be possible for totally blind people to experience visual sensations that are corticofugally constructed on the retina either during mental visual imagination or during physical brain stimulation, so long as their eyes have not been bilaterally enucleated or otherwise disconnected from the brain. One of the earliest pieces of evidence supporting this

implication comes from Charles Darwin's grandfather, Erasmus Darwin (1803), who reported that "two men, who had been some years blind; one of them had a complete gutta serena [a complete degeneration of the optic nerve], and the other man lost the whole substances of his eyes . . . told me that they did not remember ever to have dreamt of visible objects, since the total loss of their sight" (p. 15). However, two reports from eyeless persons suggest that visual sensations of redness, specifically sensations of red blood, may have accompanied their experiences of photopsia, albeit not their voluntary visual imagery nor their dream imagery other than the photopsia. The first report is described by Calderaro (1909), as translated by Shelley Berlin:

> [Despite the removal of both eyes, the 50-year-old man's photopsia continued; he noticed] a reddish colored liquid, with tone varying from light to dark red, moving continuously in waves in correspondence with the left visual field: The direction of this undulating movement is variable, being able to take place in all the senses, but the movement prevails from high to low as if the blazing liquid were flushing from the left side of the forehead. Another time, in the middle of this red liquid were perceived some sparks of a brighter red. Another time, the luminous liquid was not there and there came perception of sparks in the form of a comma or half moon. In periods of calm, the sparks assumed a whitish tint, while in periods of excitement they became a fiery bright red. Once in a great while he notices a white cloud, but for him it is mostly the color red that prevails; he does not perceive other "chromatic sensations." [The photopsy was not perceived during sleep.] (pp. 3503–3504)

The second report is described by Baquis (1932), as translated by Shelley Berlin:

> [A couple of years after the removal of the right eye and a couple of days after the operation for glaucoma in the left eye, the tormenting vision of a luminous disk appeared. Subsequent removal of the left eye did not alter this vision.] Little by little this luminous disk began to be covered with designs and swirls, like graffiti on a white wall. Between the lines of the graffiti were intersecting lines of all varied colors, like a mosaic, and blood spots at times moving about on it. . . . The bigger the disk, the clearer the designs of the graffiti. [Initially, the photopsy interfered with sleep; however, now it is possible to sleep or at least doze, even during the most intense photopsia.] (pp. 274–275)

Aside from the emotional quality of such redness, such bloodiness, what raises doubts as to whether the sensory quality of redness actually accompanied either photopsia is past research, raising doubts about the color imaging ability and tacit color knowledge of blind people. In particular, Shepard and Cooper (1992) asked totally blind persons, color-blind persons, and normally sighted persons to rank each of nine color names in between two endpoints of color, and multidimensional scaling of the rankings yielded Newton's color circle for individuals who were normally sighted or color blind, but not for individuals who were totally blind. Nevertheless, there should be no doubt as to blind people's ability to engage in imageless thinking about sensationless color-constancy features and other sensationless visual features that are represented cortically. As recent research shows, blind people's tactile and proprioceptive imaging of object form, spatial location, and human action activates sensationless visuospatial features in the same cortical regions where sensationless visuospatial features are activated by sighted people's visual imaging of object form, spatial location, and human action (Bonino et al., 2008; Cattaneo & Vecchi, 2011; Pietrini et al., 2004; Ricciardi et al., 2009). So the fact that many totally blind persons, even the congenitally blind and even the eyeless, sometimes use visual terms to describe form, location, action, and other constancies should not mislead us into concluding that their verbal descriptions reflect visually imaged sensations, as opposed to sensationless cortical knowledge and sometimes the construction of tactilely or proprioceptively imaged sensations from that knowledge.

15. I recall, as a young child, imaging so vividly that I wondered what happened to the perceptual world "blocked out" by my fantasies. So I am inclined to believe artists and other adults who report that their visual images completely or partially block out the perceptual background, even though in adulthood I can no longer image vividly enough to block out perceptual sensations. Furthermore, research findings yet to be discussed in this chapter—Doob's (1970) finding that children are four times more likely than adults to report visual images vivid enough to be "seen in front of" actual percepts, and Kunzendorf's (1989) finding that children are eight times more likely than adults to generate visual images vivid enough to induce after-sensations of fixed retinal size—are consistent with my own developmental decline in image vividness.

16. The presumption that centrifugal fibers to the human retina might serve an attentional function (rather than a developmental function as presently proposed) and the mixed evidence for this presumption have led some researchers to doubt the existence and/or the importance of such fibers (Brindley & Hamasaki, 1962; Repérant & Gallego, 1976; Repérant, Miceli, Vesselkin, & Molotchnikoff, 1989). Accordingly, in a series of studies coming out of Robert Eason's lab at the University of North Carolina in Greensboro, the b-wave of the flash electroretinogram (ERG)—the retinal response that peaks approximately 60 milliseconds after the onset of a light flash, and that increases in amplitude as the flash gets brighter (Armington, 1974)—tended to increase in amplitude also when humans selectively attended to the flash (Eason, 1984; Eason, Flowers, & Oakley, 1983; Eason, Oakley, & Flowers, 1983). In attempting to replicate Eason's results, however, Mangun, Hansen, and Hillyard (1986) from the University of California at La Jolla failed to find any effect of attention on the ERG b-wave. In March of 1991, when I went to UNC-Greensboro to give an invited research colloquium, I asked Bob Eason whether there were any individual differences in his results, and he replied that half of the subjects' ERGs exhibited attentional effects and the other half's ERGs exhibited no effects of attention. In normal subjects, one wouldn't expect to find individual differences in attentional gating. But if one were to think about attention not in terms of neurological gating, but in terms of anticipatory imaging, as in Kingsley's (1932) approach to attention, then one might sensibly conclude that individual differences in attention reflect individual differences in imaging ability. Such an approach has been adopted in recent times only by researchers studying "search images" in predatory animals, some of whom also study the centrifugal nature of such images, as we shall soon see.

17. Whether or not this source-verifying information gets encoded in memory is an interesting empirical question, given Marcia Johnson's (1988, 1991) evidence that many people misremember previously imaged experiences as previously perceived experiences. Such "false memory" for previously imaged experiences has been found to be positively correlated with greater image vividness (Dobson & Markham, 1993; Horselenberg et al., 2000; Hyman & Billings, 1998; Kunzendorf, Deignan, Galva, Latorre, & Masotta, 2005–2006; Markham & Hynes, 1993; Niedźwieńska, 2000–2001), uncorrelated with image vividness (Aleman & de Haan, 2004; Belliveau & Kunzendorf (2014–2015; Candel, Merckelbach, & Kuijpers, 2003; Chang, 2008; Drivdahl & Zaragoza, 2001; Heaps & Nash, 1999; Paddock et al., 1999; Wilkinson & Hyman, 1998) and negatively correlated with greater image vividness (Horselenberg, Merckelbach, van Breukelen, & Wessel, 2004; Kunzendorf, 1992–1993). In the only study controlling both for response biases and for inter-correlations, Belliveau and Kunzendorf (2014–2015) found that false memory was positively correlated with dissociative amnesia, but uncorrelated with image vividness. The current chapter is focused on immediate reality-testing or self-conscious source verification in real time, however, and is not concerned with memory for source.
18. In relation to the seemingly unconscious percepts of patients with lesions in area V1 (i.e., patients with "blindsight"), Thomas Natsoulas (2000–2001) suggests that such percepts might also be conscious sensations that are unaccompanied by self-consciousness that *one is perceiving*. Indeed, consistent with Natsoulas's suggestion, Lawrence Weiskrantz (2002) discovered that, even though his blindsighted patients do not experience percepts in their cortically blind field of vision, they do experience afterimages or after-sensations of those percepts. To date, however, research has not tested whether blindsighted persons are simply unable to self-consciously verify the perceptual source of their perceived sensations while they are actively perceiving those sensations in real time.
19. Children's source-memory for distinguishing their previously performed actions, their previously pretended actions, and their previously imagined actions doesn't plateau until a few years later (Foley & Johnson, 1985; Roberts & Blades, 1995; Welch-Ross, 1995).
20. Research summarized by Kunzendorf (2007c) shows how visual images, in the context of lingering emotions, tend to give visual expression to those emotions (Hartmann & Kunzendorf, 2005-2006; Hartmann et al., 2002–2003; Hartmann, Kunzendorf, Rosen, & Grace, 2001; Hartmann, Zborowski, & Kunzendorf, 2001; Hartmann, Zborowski, Rosen, & Grace, 2001; Kunzendorf, Hartmann, Thomas, & Berensen, 1999–2000).
21. It is noteworthy that Kunzendorf, Crosson, Zalaket, White, and Enik (1998-1999) developed a questionnaire to score the three diagnostic criteria for Dissociative Identity Disorder in DSM-VI (American Psychiatric Association, 1994) and discovered that college students' scores on two of the scaled criteria—"multiple self-identities" and "multiple self-controls"—were normally distributed and were associated with the nonpathological "absorption in fantasy" factor on Bernstein and Putnam's (1986) Dissociative Experiences Scale (DES). Only scores on the third criterion—"recall amnesia/source amnesia"—were skewed in the direction of higher scores and were statistically associated with the two DES factors indicative of pathological dissociation.

References

Abdolmaleky, H. M., Cheng, K.-H., Faraone, S. V., Wilcox, M., Glatt, S. J., Gao, F., et al. (2006). Hypomethylation of MB-COMT promoter is a major risk factor for schizophrenia and bipolar disorder. *Human Molecular Genetics, 15,* 3132–3145.

Al-Anzi, B., Tracey, W. D., Jr., & Benzer, S. (2006). Response of *Drosophila* to wasabi is mediated by *painless,* the fly homolog of mammalian TRPA1/ANKTM1. *Current Biology, 16,* 1034–1040.

Aleman, A., Böcker, K. B. E., Hijman, R., de Haan, E. H. F., & Kahn, R. S. (2003). Cognitive basis of hallucinations in schizophrenia: Role of top-down information processing. *Schizophrenia Research, 64,* 175–185.

Aleman, A., & de Haan, E. H. F. (2004). Fantasy proneness, mental imagery and reality monitoring. *Personality and Individual Differences, 36,* 1747–1754.

Allen, J. G., Coyne, L., & Console, D. A. (1997). Dissociative detachment relates to psychotic symptoms and personality decompensation. *Comprehensive Psychiatry, 38,* 327–334.

Alloy, L. B., & Abramson, L. (1979). Judgement of contingency in depressed and non-depressed students: Sadder but wiser? *Journal of Experimental Psychology: General, 108,* 441–485.

Alloy, L. B., & Abramson, L. (1988). Depressive realism: Four theoretical perspectives. In L. B. Alloy (Ed.), *Cognitive processes in depression* (pp. 223–265). New York, NY: Guilford.

American Psychiatric Association. (1994). *Diagnostic and statistical manual of mental disorders* (4th ed.). Washington, DC: American Psychiatric Association.

Animal Life Resource. (2012a). *Anemones and corals: Anthozoa—Behavior and reproduction.* Retrieved from http://animals.jrank.org/pages/1471/Anemones-Corals-Anthozoa-BEHAVIOR-REPRODUCTION.html

Animal Life Resource. (2012b). *Jellyfish: Scyphozoa—Behavior and reproduction.* Retrieved from http://animals.jrank.org/pages/1491/Jellyfish-Scyphozoa-BEHAVIOR-REPRODUCTION.html

Antonietti, A., Bologna, D., & Lupi, G. (1997). Creative synthesis of visual images is not associated with individual differences. *Perceptual and Motor Skills, 85,* 881–882.

Armington, J. C. (1974). *The electroretinogram.* New York, NY: Academic.

Arnheim, R. (1969). *Visual thinking.* Berkeley, CA: University of California Press.

Arseneault, L., Moffitt, T. E., Caspi, A., Taylor, P. J., & Silva, P. A. (2000). Mental disorders and violence in a total birth cohort: Results from the Dunedin study. *Archives of General Psychiatry, 57,* 979–986.

Aserinsky, E., & Kleitman, N. (1955). Two types of ocular motility occurring in sleep. *Journal of Applied Physiology, 8,* 1–10.

Ashton, R., McFarland, K., Walsh, F., & White, K. (1978). Imagery ability and the identification of hands: A chronometric analysis. *Acta Psychologica, 42,* 253–262.

Baars, B. J. (1988). *A cognitive theory of consciousness.* New York, NY: Cambridge University Press.

Bain, A. (1868). *Mental science: A compendium of psychology, and the history of philosophy.* New York, NY: Appleton.

Bandah, D., Swissa, T., Ben-Shlomo, G., Banin, E., Ofri, R., & Sharon, D. (2007). A complex expression pattern of *Pax6* in the pigeon retina. *Investigative Ophthalmology & Visual Science, 48,* 2503–2509.

Baquis, M. (1932). Fotopsia ed allucinazioni visive negli individui privi di ambedue gli occhi. *Lettura Oftalmologica, 9,* 271–281.

Barber, T. X. (1984). Changing "unchangeable" bodily processes by (hypnotic) suggestions: A new look at hypnosis, cognitions, imagining and the mind-body problem. *Advances, 1,* 7–40.

Bard, P., & Roich, D. M. (1937). A study of four cats deprived of neocortex and additional portions of the forebrain. *Bulletin of the Johns Hopkins Hospital, 60,* 73–148.

Barrett, D. (1992). Just how lucid are lucid dreams? *Dreaming, 2,* 221–228.

Barrett, D. (2001). *The committee of sleep: How artists, scientists, and athletes use dreams for creative problem-solving—and how you can too.* Norwalk, CT: Crown House.

Baust, W., Berlucchi, G., & Moruzzi, G. (1964). Changes in the auditory input in wakefulness and during the synchronized and desynchronized stages of sleep. *Archives Italiennes de Biologie, 102,* 657–674.

Baylor, D. A., Lamb, T. D., & Yau, K.-W. (1979). Responses of retinal rods to single photons. *Journal of Physiology, 288,* 613–634.

Becker, E. (1973). *The denial of death.* New York, NY: Free Press.

Becker, E. (1975). *Escape from evil.* New York, NY: Free Press.

Beirens, K., & Fontaine, J. R. J. (2010). Validity of the Ghent Multidimensional Somatic Complaint Scale in a clinical population. *Journal of Psychosomatic Research, 68,* 535-538.

Belliveau, D., & Kunzendorf, R. G. (2014–2015). Is forced-choice false recognition associated with image vividness, dissociative factors, or their interaction? *Imagination, Cognition, and Personality, 34,* 218-229.

Belluck, P., & Carey, B. (2013, May 7). Psychiatry's new guide falls short, experts say. *New York Times,* pp. A12, A15.

Belousova, T. A., Devitsina, G. V., & Malyukina, G. A. (1983). Functional peculiarities of fish trigeminal system. *Chemical Senses, 8,* 121–130.

Bender, M. B., Shapiro, M. F., & Teuber, H.-L. (1949). Allesthesia and disturbance of the body scheme. *Archives of Neurology & Psychiatry, 62,* 222–235.

Benedetti, F., Dallaspezia, S., Colombo, C., Lorenzi, C., Pirovano, A., & Smeraldi, E. (2010). Association between Catechol-O-methyltransferase Val(108/158)Met polymorphism and psychotic features of bipolar disorder. *Journal of Affective Disorders, 125,* 341–344.

Berstrin, D. P., Stein, J. A., Newcomb, M. D., Walker, E., Pogge, D., Ahluvalia, T., et al. (2003). Development and validation of a brief screening version of the Childhood Trauma Questionnaire. *Child Abuse & Neglect, 27*, 169-190.

Bernstein, E. M., & Putnam, F. W. (1986). Development, reliability, and validity of a dissociation scale. *Journal of Nervous and Mental Disease, 174,* 727–735.

Bethel-Fox, C. E., Lohman, D. F., & Snow, R. E. (1984). Adaptive reasoning: Componential and eye movement analysis of geometric analogy performance. *Intelligence, 8,* 205–238.

Betts, G. H. (1909). *The distribution and functions of mental imagery.* New York, NY: Teachers College, Columbia University.

Bhatnagar, S. C., Andy, O. J., & Linville, S. (1989). Tonotypic cortical representation in man. *Pavlovian Journal of Biological Science, 24,* 50–53.

Bittini, M., & Ronchi, L. (1958). May psychological factors influence the electroretinographic response? *Atti della Fondazione Giorgo Ronchi, 12,* 417–418.

Blackmore, S. (2004). *Consciousness: An introduction.* New York, NY: Oxford University Press.

Blackshaw, S. E., Nicholls, J. G., & Parnas, I. (1982). Expanded receptive fields of cutaneous mechanoreceptor cells after single neurone deletion in leech central nervous system. *Journal of Physiology, 326,* 261–268.

Bliss, E. (1986). *Multiple personality, allied disorders, and hypnosis.* New York, NY: Oxford University Press.

Bloch, M. N., & Adler, S. M. (1994). African children's play and the emergence of the sexual division of labor. In J. L. Roopnarine, J. E. Johnson, & F. H. Hooper (Eds.), *Children's play in diverse cultures* (pp. 148–178). Albany, NY: State University of New York.

Böcker, K. B. E., Hijman, R., Kahn, R. S., & de Haan, E. H. F. (2000). Perception, mental imagery and reality discrimination in hallucinating and non-hallucinating schizophrenic patients. *British Journal of Clinical Psychology, 39,* 397–406.

Bogoslovskii, A., & Semenovskaya, E. (1959). Conditioned reflex changes in the human electroretinogram. *Bulletin of Experimental Biology and Medicine, 47,* 265–269.

Bolanowski, S. J., Gescheider, G. A., Verrillo, R. T., & Checkosky, C. M. (1988). Four channels mediate the mechanical aspects of touch. *Journal of the Acoustical Society of America, 84,* 1680–1694.

Bonino, D., Ricciardi, E., Sani, L., Gentili, C., Vanello, N., Guazzelli, M., et al. (2008). Tactile spatial working memory activates the dorsal extrastriate cortical pathway in congenitally blind individuals. *Archives Italiennes de Biologie, 146,* 133–146.

Boord, R. L. (1961). The efferent cochlear bundle in the caiman and pigeon. *Experimental Neurology, 3,* 225–239.

Boring, E. G. (1929). *A history of experimental psychology*. New York, NY: Appleton-Century.

Bowers, H. (1935). The role of visual imagery in reasoning. *British Journal of Psychology, 25,* 436–446.

Bowmaker, J. K. (2008). Evolution of vertebrate visual pigments. *Vision Research, 48,* 2022–2041.

Bradshaw, I. G. A. (2004). Not by bread alone: Symbolic loss, trauma, and recovery in elephant communities. *Society & Animals, 12,* 143–158.

Brainerd, C. J. (1971). The development of the proportionality scheme in children and adolescents. *Developmental Psychology, 5,* 469–476.

Brennan, P. A., Mednick, S. A., & Hodgins, S. (2000). Major mental disorders and criminal violence in a Danish birth cohort. *Archives of General Psychiatry, 57,* 494–500.

Brett, E. A., & Starker, S. (1977). Auditory imagery and hallucinations. *Journal of Nervous and Mental Disease, 164,* 394–400.

Breugelmans, S. M., Ambadar, Z., Vaca, J. B., Poortinga, Y. H., Setiadi, B., Widiyanto, P., & Philippot, P. (2005). Body sensations associated with emotions in Rarámuri Indians, rural Javaneses, and three student samples. *Emotion, 5,* 166-174.

Brindley, G. S., & Hamasaki, D. I. (1962). Evidence that the cat's electroretinogram is not influenced by impulses passing to the eye along the optic nerve. *Journal of Physiology, 163,* 558–565.

Briñón, J. G., Crespo, C., Weruaga, E., Alonso, J., Sobreviela, T., Aijón, J., & Alonso, J. R. (1998). NADPH-diaphorase/nitric oxide synthase-positive elements in the human olfactory bulb. *Neuroreport, 9,* 3141–3146.

Broackes, J. (2010). What do the color-blind see? In J. Cohen & M. Matthen (Eds.), *Color ontology and color science* (pp. 291–405). Cambridge, MA: MIT Press.

Broesch, T., Callaghan, T., Henrich, J., Murphy, C., & Rochat, P. (2011). Cultural variations in children's mirror self-recognition. *Journal of Cross-Cultural Psychology, 42,* 1018–1029.

Brooks, E. M. (2004–2005). Multiplicity of consciousness. *Imagination, Cognition and Personality, 24,* 271–280.

Brooks, E. M. (2011–2012). Ontology theory of consciousness. *Imagination, Cognition and Personality, 31,* 217–235.

Brown, G. E., & Stroup, K. (1988). Learned helplessness in the cockroach (Periplaneta Americana). *Behavioral & Neural Biology, 50,* 246–250.

Budelmann, B. U. (1992). Hearing in nonarthropod invertebrates. In D. B. Webster, R. R. Fay, & A. N. Popper (Eds.), *The evolutionary biology of hearing* (pp. 141–155). New York, NY: Springer-Verlag.

Bühler, K. (1964). Thinking and the new psychology: Imageless thought. In J. M. Mandler & G. Mandler (Eds. & Trans.), *Thinking: From association to Gestalt* (pp. 162–164). New York, NY: John Wiley. (Original 1907 article published in German in *Archiv für die Gesamte Psychologie, 9,* 297–365)

Bull, H. O. (1928). Studies on conditioned responses in fishes. Part I. *Journal of the Marine Biological Association of the United Kingdom, 15,* 485–533.

Bull, H. O. (1935). Studies on conditioned responses in fishes. 3. Wave length discrimination in Blennius pholis L. *Journal of the Marine Biological Association of the United Kingdom, 20,* 347–364.

Byrne, J. H., & Crow, T. (1991). Examples of mechanistic analyses of learning and memory in invertebrates. In J. L. Martinez & R. P. Kesner (Eds.), *Learning and memory: A biological view* (pp. 329–358). San Diego, CA: Academic.

Calderaro, S. (1909). Fotopsie in individui privi di globi oculari. *La Clinica Oculistica, 10,* 3501–3513.

Campbell, C. A. (1957). *On selfhood and godhood.* New York, NY: Macmillan.

Candel, I., Merckelbach, H., & Kuijpers, M. (2003). Dissociative experiences are related to commissions in emotional memory. *Behaviour Research and Therapy, 41,* 719–725.

Capellini, I. (2012). Phylogeny of sleep. In D. Barrett & P. McNamara (Eds.), *Encyclopedia of sleep and dreams: The evolution, function, nature, and mysteries of slumber* (Vol. 2, pp. 497–504). Santa Barbara, CA: Greenwood.

Cardno, A. G., Rijsdijk, F. V., Sham, P. C. Murray, R. M., & McGuffin, P. (2002). A twin study of genetic relationships between psychotic symptoms. *American Journal of Psychiatry, 159,* 539–545.

Cattaneo, Z., & Vecchi, T. (2011). *Blind vision.* Cambridge, MA: MIT Press.

Chandiramani, K., & Varma, V. K. (1987). Imagery in schizophrenic patients compared with normal controls. *British Journal of Medical Psychology, 60,* 335–341.

Chang, S. H. (2008). Individual differences in imagery ability on false memories. *Dissertation Abstracts International: Section B: The Sciences and Engineering, 68,* 4854.

Chapman, M. (1987). A longitudinal study of cognitive representation in symbolic play, self-recognition, and object permanence during the second year. *International Journal of Behavioral Development, 10,* 151–170.

Chase, R., & Tolloczko, B. (1993). Tracing neural pathways in snail olfaction: From the tip of the tentacles to the brain and beyond. *Microscopy Research and Technique, 24,* 214–230.

Chen, Q.-Y., Alarcon, S., Tharp, A., Ahmed, O. M., Estrella, N. L., Greene, T. A., Rucker, J., & Breslin, P. A. S. (2009). Perceptual variation in umami taste and polymorphisms in TAS1R taste receptor genes. *American Journal of Clinical Nutrition, 90,* 770S–779S.

Chen, W., Kato, T., Zhu, X.-H., Ogawa, S., Rank, D. W., & Ugurbil, K. (1998). Human primary visual cortex and lateral geniculate nucleus activation during visual imagery. *Neuroreport: An International Journal for the Rapid Communication of Research in Neuroscience, 9,* 3669–3674.

Chomsky, N. (1968). *Language and mind.* New York, NY: Harcourt, Brace & World.

Clarke, R. W., Wych, B. E., & Harris, J. (2001). Adaptive changes in withdrawal reflexes after noxious stimulation at the heel and the toes in the decerebrated rabbit. *Neuroscience Letters, 304,* 120–122.

Cohen, B. D., & Camhi, J. (1967). Schizophrenic performance in a word-communication task. *Journal of Abnormal Psychology, 72,* 240–246.

Cohen, B. D., Nachmani, G., & Rosenberg, S. (1974). Referent communication disturbances in acute schizophrenia. *Journal of Abnormal Psychology, 83,* 1–13.

Cohen, Y., Reuveni, I., Barkai, E., & Maroun, M. (2008). Olfactory learning-induced long-lasting enhancement of descending and ascending synaptic transmission to the piriform cortex. *Journal of Neuroscience, 28,* 6664–6669.

Cooper, K. K. (1972). Cutaneous mechanoreceptors of the glans penis of the cat. *Physiology and Behavior, 8,* 793–796.

Corteen, R. S., & Wood, B. (1972). Autonomic responses to shock-associated words in an unattended channel. *Journal of Experimental Psychology, 94,* 308–313.

Coryell, W., Pfohl, B., & Zimmerman, M. (1984). The clinical and neuroendocrine features of psychotic depression. *Journal of Nervous and Mental Disease, 172,* 521–528.

Costafreda, S. G., Brébion, G., Allen, P., McGuire, P. K., & Fu, C. H. Y. (2008). Affective modulation of external misattribution bias in source monitoring in schizophrenia. *Psychological Medicine, 38,* 821–824.

Cox, M. (2005). *The pictorial world of the child.* Cambridge, UK: Cambridge University Press.

Crick, F. (1994). *The astonishing hypothesis: The scientific search for the soul*. New York, NY: Simon & Schuster.

Cronholm, B. (1951). Phantom limbs in amputees: A study in changes in the integration of centripetal impulses with special reference to referred sensations. *Acta Psychiatrica et Neurologica, 72*(Suppl.), 7–310.

D'Angiulli, A. (2002). Mental image generation and the contrast sensitivity function. *Cognition, 85,* B11–B19.

Darwin, C. (1859). *On the origin of species by means of natural selection*. London, UK: John Murray.

Darwin, C. (2007). *The descent of man*. London, UK: Penguin. (Original work published 1871, rev. 1879)

Darwin, C. (2009). *The expression of the emotions in man and animals, 200th anniversary edition, Charles Darwin 1809–1882* (P. Ekman, Ed.). Oxford, UK: Oxford University Press. (Original work published 1872)

Darwin, E. (1803). *Zoonomia* (Vol. 1). Boston, MA: D. Carlisle.

Davidson, C., Prados, J., Gibson, C. L., Young, A. M. J., Barnes, D., Sherlock, R., & Hutchinson, C. V. (2011). Shedding light on photosensitive behaviour in brown planaria (*Dugesia Tigrina*). *Perception, 40,* 743–746.

Davis, K. D., Kiss, Z. H. T., Tasker, R. R., & Dostrovsky, J. O. (1996). Thalamic stimulation-evoked sensations in chronic pain patients and in nonpain (movement disorder) patients. *Journal of Neurophysiology, 75,* 1026–1037.

Dean, G., & Morris, P. E. (1991). Imagery and spatial ability: When introspective reports predict performance. In R. H. Logie & M. Denis (Eds.), *Mental images in human cognition* (pp. 331–347). Amsterdam, The Netherlands: Elsevier.

de Bono, M., & Maricq, A. V. (2005). Neural substrates of complex behaviors in *C. elegans*. *Annual Review of Neuroscience, 28,* 451–501.

Dehon, H., Bastin, C., & Larøi, F. (2008). The influence of delusional ideation and dissociative experiences on the resistance to false memories in normal healthy subjects. *Personality and Individual Differences, 45,* 62–67.

Delfour, F., & Marten, K. (2001). Mirror image processing in three marine mammal species: Killer whales (*Orcinus orca*), false killer whales (*Pseudorca crassidents*) and California sea lions (*Zalophus californianus*). *Behavioural Processes, 53,* 181–190.

De Luca, C. R., & Leventer, R. J. (2008). Developmental trajectories of executive functions across the lifespan. In V. Anderson, R. Jacobs, & P. J. Anderson (Eds.), *Executive functions and the frontal lobes: A lifespan perspective* (pp. 23–56). New York, NY: Taylor & Francis.

Dement, W., & Kleitman, N. (1957). The relation of eye movements during sleep to dream activity: An objective method for the study of dreaming. *Journal of Experimental Psychology, 53,* 339–346.

Dennett, D. C. (1991). *Consciousness explained*. Boston, MA: Little Brown.

Denny-Brown, D. (1966). *The cerebral control of movement*. Liverpool, UK: Liverpool University Press.

Denton, D. A., McKinley, M. J., Farrell, M., & Egan, G. F. (2009). The role of primordial emotions in the evolutionary origin of consciousness. *Consciousness and Cognition, 18,* 500–514.

DeRosse, P., Malhotra, A. K., & Lencz, T. (2012). Molecular genetics of the psychosis phenotype. *Psychosis, 57,* 446–453.

Descartes, R. (1988). The existence of material things: The real distinction between mind and body [an adaptation of *Meditationes de prima philosophia*, originally published in 1641, translated by E. S. Haldane & G. R. T. Ross and republished by Cambridge University Press in 1911]. In L. T. Benjamin, Jr. (Ed.), *A history of psychology: Original sources and contemporary research* (pp. 36–43). New York, NY: McGraw-Hill.

Desmedt, J. E. (1962). Auditory-evoked potentials from cochlea to cortex as influenced by activation of the efferent olivocochlear bundle. *Journal of the Acoustical Society of America, 34,* 1478–1496.

Devor, M. (2006). Response of nerves to injury in relation to neuropathic pain. In S. L. McMahon & M. Koltzenburg (Eds.), *Wall and Melzack's textbook of pain* (5th ed., pp. 905–927). London, UK: Churchill Livingston.

Devor, M. (2007). Pain, cortex, and consciousness. *Behavioural and Brain Sciences, 30,* 89–90.

Devor, M. (2009). Nerves hurt. *European Journal of Pain, 13,* 1–2.

DiVesta, F. J., Ingersoll, G., & Sunshine, P. (1971). A factor analysis of imagery tests. *Journal of Verbal Learning and Verbal Behavior, 10,* 471–479.

Dixon, N. F. (1971). *Subliminal perception*. London, UK: McGraw-Hill.

Dixon. N. F. (1981). *Preconscious processing*. Chichester, UK: John Wiley.

Dobson, M., & Markham, R. (1993). Imagery ability and source monitoring: Implications for eyewitness memory. *British Journal of Psychology, 84,* 111–118.

Dodt, E. (1956). Centrifugal impulses in rabbit's retina. *Journal of Neurophysiology, 19,* 301–307.

Doob, L. W. (1970). Correlates of mental imagery in Africa. *Journal of Psychology: Interdisciplinary and Applied, 76,* 223–230.

Dostrovsky, J. O., Davis, K. D., Lee, L., Sher, G. D., & Tasker, R. R. (1993). Electrical stimulation-induced effects in the human thalamus. In O. Devinsky, A. Berić, & M. Dogali (Eds.), *Electrical and magnetic stimulation of the brain and spinal cord* (pp. 219–229. New York, NY: Raven.

Drivdahl, S. B., & Zaragoza, M. S. (2001). The role of perceptual elaboration and individual differences in the creation of false memories for suggested events. *Applied Cognitive Psychology, 15,* 265–281.

Duffy, K. R., & Hubel, D. H. (2007). Receptive field properties of neurons in the primary visual cortex under photopic and scotopic lighting conditions. *Vision Research, 47,* 2569–2574.

Durier, V., & Rivault, C. (2001). Effects of spatial knowledge and feeding experience on foraging choices in German cockroaches. *Animal Behaviour, 62,* 681–688.

Durndell, A. J., & Wetherick, N. E. (1976). Reported imagery and two spatial tests. *Perceptual and Motor Skills, 43,* 1050.

Eason, R. G. (1984). Selective attention effects on retinal and forebrain responses in humans: A replication and extension. *Bulletin of the Psychonomic Society, 22,* 341–344.

Eason, R. G., Flowers, L., & Oakley, M. (1983). Differentiation of retinal and non-retinal contributions to averaged evoked responses obtained with electrodes placed near the eyes. *Behavior Research Methods & Instrumentation, 15,* 13–21.

Eason, R. G., Oakley, M., & Flowers, L. (1983). Central neural influences on the human retina during selective attention. *Physiological Psychology, 11,* 18–28.

Eberl, D. F., Hardy, R. W., & Kernan, M. J. (2000). Genetically similar transduction mechanisms for touch and hearing in *Drosophila. Journal of Neuroscience, 20,* 5981–5988.

Eccles, J. C. (1988). The spiritual nature of the self. *Dynamische Psychiatrie, 21,* 20–34.

Elkin-Frankston, S., Fried, P. J., Pascual-Leone, A., Rushmore, R. J., III, & Valero-Cabr, A. (2010). A novel approach for documenting phosphenes induced by transcranial magnetic stimulation. *Journal of Visualized Experiments, 38,* 1762–1765.

Fechner, G. T. (1966). *Elements of psychophysics* (H. E. Adler, Trans.). New York, NY: Holt, Rinehart, and Winston. (Original work published 1860)

Feigl, H. (1958). The "mental" and the "physical." *Minnesota Studies in the Philosophy of Science, 2,* 370–497.

Feinle, C. (1998). Role of intestinal chemoreception in the induction of gastrointestinal sensations. *Deutsche tierärztliche Wochenschrift, 105,* 441–444.

Ferrari, M., & Matthews, W. S. (1983). Self-recognition deficits in autism: Syndrome-specific or general developmental delay? *Journal of Autism and Developmental Disorders, 13,* 317–324.

Fex, J. (1959). Augmentation of cochlear microphonic by stimulation of efferent fibres to the cochlea. *Acta Oto-Laryngologica, 50,* 540–541.

Fletcher, P., Büchel, C., Josephs, O., Friston, K., & Dolan, R. (1999). Learning-related neuronal responses in prefrontal cortex studied with functional neuroimaging. *Cerebral Cortex, 9,* 168–178.

Fodor, J. A. (1968). The appeal to tacit knowledge in psychological explanation. *Journal of Philosophy, 65,* 627–640.

Foley, M. A., & Johnson, M. K. (1985). Confusions between memories for performed and imagined actions: A developmental comparison. *Child Development, 56,* 1145–1155.

Fountain, S. B. (2008). Pattern structure and rule induction in sequential learning. *Comparative Cognition & Behavior Review, 3,* 66–85.

Freedman, S. J., & Ronchi, L. (1964). Adaptation and training effects in ERG: IV. Overview of eight years. *Atti della Fondazione Giorgo Ronchi, 19,* 542–565.

Freeman, W. J. (1983). The physiological basis of mental images. *Biological Psychiatry, 18,* 1107–1125.

Freud, S. (1924). *A general introduction to psychoanalysis* (J. Riviere, Trans.). New York, NY: Boni and Liveright.

Fujita, I., Satou, M., & Ueda, K. (1984). A field-potential study of centripetal and centrifugal connections of the olfactory bulb in the carp, Cuprinus carpio (L.). *Brain Research, 32,* 33–44.

Fuster, J. M. (2000). The prefrontal cortex of the primate: A synopsis. *Psychobiology, 28,* 125–131.

Gacek, R. R. (1961). The efferent cochlear bundle in man. *Archives of Otolaryngology, 74,* 690–694.

Galambos, R. (1956). Suppression of auditory nerve activity by stimulation of efferent fibers to cochlea. *Journal of Neurophysiology, 19,* 424–437.

Galambos, R., Szabó-Salfay, O., Szatmári, E., Szilágyi, N., & Juhász, G. (2001). Sleep modifies retinal ganglion cell responses in the normal rat. *Proceedings of the National Academy of Sciences, 98,* 2083–2088.

Gallup, G. G., Jr. (1968). Mirror-image stimulation. *Psychological Bulletin, 70,* 782–793.

Gallup, G. G., Jr. (1970). Chimpanzees: Self-recognition. *Science, 167,* 86–87.

Gallup, G. G., Jr. (1977). Self-recognition in primates: A comparative approach to the bidirectional properties of consciousness. *American Psychologist, 32,* 329–338.

Gallup, G. G., Jr. (1979). Self-awareness in primates. *American Scientist, 67,* 417–421.

Gallup, G. G., Jr., Anderson, J. R., & Platek, S. M. (2003). Self-awareness, social intelligence and schizophrenia. In T. Kircher & A. David (Eds.), *The self in neuroscience and psychiatry* (pp. 147–165). New York, NY: Cambridge University Press.

Geary, D. C. (2009). The evolution of general fluid intelligence. In S. M. Platek & T. K. Shackelford (Eds.), *Foundations in evolutionary cognitive neuroscience* (pp. 22–56). Cambridge, UK: Cambridge University Press.

Gehring, W. J. (1996). The master control gene for morphogenesis and evolution of the eye. *Genes to Cells, 1,* 11–15.

Gentner, T. Q., Fenn, K. M., Margoliash, D., & Nusbaum, H. C. (2006). Recursive syntactic pattern learning by songbirds. *Nature, 440,* 1204–1207.

German, T. P., Niehaus, J. L., Roarty, M. P., Giesbrecht, B., & Miller, M. B. (2004). Neural correlates of detecting pretense: Automatic engagement of the intentional stance under covert conditions. *Journal of Cognitive Neuroscience, 16,* 1805–1817.

Giambra, L. M. (2000). Daydreaming characteristics across the life-span: Age differences and seven to twenty year longitudinal changes. In R. G. Kunzendorf & B. Wallace (Eds.), *Individual differences in conscious experience* (pp. 147–206). Amsterdam, The Netherlands: John Benjamins.

Gimranov, R. F. (2004). Changes in bioelectric activity in the human retina after transcranial magnetic stimulation. *Human Physiology, 30,* 47–49.

Giurfa, M., & Sandoz, J.-C. (2012). Invertebrate learning and memory: Fifty years of olfactory conditioning of the proboscis extension response in honeybees. *Learning & Memory, 19,* 54–66.

Goghari, V. M., & Sponheim, S. R. (2008). Differential association of the COMT Val158Met polymorphism with clinical phenotypes in schizophrenia and bipolar disorder. *Schizophrenia Research, 103,* 186–191.

Goodnow, J. J., & Friedman, S. (1972). Orientation in children's human figure drawings: An aspect of graphic language. *Developmental Psychology, 7,* 10–16.

Goodwin, S. J., Blackman, R. K., Sakellaridi, S., & Chafee, M. V. (2012). Executive control over cognition: Stronger and earlier rule-based modulation of spatial category signals in prefrontal cortex relative to parietal cortex. *Journal of Neuroscience, 32,* 3499–3515.

Granit, R. (1955). Centrifugal and antidromic effects on ganglion cells of retina. *Journal of Neurophysiology, 18,* 388–411.

Granrud, C. E. (2009). Development of size constancy in children: A test of the metacognitive theory. *Attention, Perception, & Psychophysics, 71,* 644–654.

Gray, J. A. (1970). The mind-brain identity theory as a scientific hypothesis. *Philosophical Quarterly, 21*, 247–254.

Greenwald, A. G. (1988). Self-knowledge and self-deception. In J. S. Lockard & D. L. Paulhus (Eds.), *Self-deception: An adaptive mechanism?* (pp. 113–131). Englewood Cliffs, NJ: Prentice Hall.

Güntürkün, O. (2005). Avian and mammalian “prefrontal cortices”: Limited degrees of freedom in the evolution of the neural mechanisms of goal-state maintenance. *Brain Research Bulletin, 66,* 311–316.

Güntürkün, O. (2012). The convergent evolution of neural substrates for cognition. *Psychological Research, 76,* 212–219.

Gupta, A. S., van der Meer, M. A. A., Touretzky, D. S., & Redish, A. D. (2010). Hippocampal replay is not a simple function of experience. *Neuron, 65,* 695–705.

Hahmann, U., & Güntürkün, O. (1992). Visual-discrimination deficits after lesions of the centrifugal visual system in pigeons (Columba livia). *Visual Neuroscience, 9,* 225–233.

Haight, W. L., Wang, X., Fung, H. H., Williams, K., & Mintz, J. (1999). Universal, developmental, and variable aspects of young children’s play: A cross-cultural comparison of pretending at home. *Child Development, 70,* 1477–1488.

Hartmann, E. (1995) Making connections in a safe place: Is dreaming psychotherapy? *Dreaming, 5,* 213–228.

Hartmann, E., Bernstein, J., & Wilson, C. (1968). Sleep + dreaming in the elephant. *Psychophysiology, 4,* 389.

Hartmann, E., & Kunzendorf, R. G. (2005–2006). The central image (CI) in recent dreams, dreams that stand out, and earliest dreams: Relationships to boundaries. *Imagination, Cognition and Personality, 25,* 383–392.

Hartmann, E., Kunzendorf, R. G., Baddour, A., Chapwick, M., Eddins, M., Krueger, C., Latraverso, T., & Shannon, R. (2002–2003). Emotion makes daydreams more dreamlike more symbolic. *Imagination, Cognition and Personality, 22,* 255–274.

Hartmann, E., Kunzendorf, R. G., Rosen, R., & Grace, N. (2001). Contextualizing images in dreams and daydreams. *Dreaming, 11,* 97–104.

Hartmann, E., Zborowski, M., & Kunzendorf, R. (2001). The emotion pictured by a dream. *Sleep and Hypnosis, 3,* 33–43.

Hartmann, E., Zborowski, M., Rosen, R., & Grace, N. (2001). Contextualizing images in dreams: More intense after abuse and trauma. *Dreaming, 11,* 115–126.

Hatakeyama, T. (1981). Individual differences in imagery ability and mental rotation. *Tohoku Psychologica Folia, 40*(1[Suppl. 4]), 6–23.

Hayes, C. (1951). *The ape in our house.* New York, NY: Harper.

Heaps, C., & Nash, M. (1999). Individual differences in imagination inflation. *Psychonomic Bulletin & Review, 6,* 313–318.

Herbranson, W. T., & Shimp, C. P. (2003). “Artificial grammar learning” in pigeons: A preliminary analysis. *Learning & Behavior, 31,* 98–106.

Herbranson, W. T., & Shimp, C. P. (2008). Artificial grammar learning in pigeons. *Learning & Behavior, 36,* 116–137.

Herman, L. M., Richards, D. G., & Wolz, J. P. (1984). Comprehensions of sentences by bottlenosed dolphins. *Cognition, 16,* 129–219.

Hernández-Peón, R., Lavin, A., Alcocer-Cuarón, C., & Marcelin, J. P. (1960). Electrical activity of the olfactory bulb during wakefulness and sleep. *Electroencephalography and Clinical Neurophysiology, 12,* 41–58.

Hernández-Peón, R., Scherrer, H., & Velasco, M. (1956). Central influences on afferent conduction in the somatic and visual pathways. *Acta Neurólogica Latinoamericana, 2,* 8–22.

Heywood, C. A., & Kentridge, R. W. (2003). Achromatopsia, color vision, and cortex. *Neurologic Clinics, 21,* 483–500.

Hilgard, E. R. (1977). *Divided consciousness: Multiple controls in human thought and action.* New York, NY: John Wiley.

Hilgard, E. R. (1981). Imagery and imagination in American psychology. *Journal of Mental Imagery, 5*(1), 5–66.

Hisata, Y., Zeredo, J. L., Eishi, K., & Toda, K. (2006). Cardiac nociceptors innervated by vagal afferents in rats. *Autonomic Neuroscience: Basic & Clinical, 126–127,* 174–178.

Hoekenga, C. (2012). Jellyfish romance—*(Carybdea sivickisi). Smithsonian Institution.* Retrieved from http://invertebrates.si.edu/jellyfish

Hofer, H., singer, B., & Williams, D. R. (2005). Different sensations from cones with the same photopigment. *Journal of Vision, 5,* 444–454.

Høffding, H. (1896). *Outlines of psychology* (M. E. Lowndes, Trans.). London, UK: Macmillan. (Original work published 1891 in Danish)

Hoffmann, T., Sauer, S. K., Horch, R. E., & Reeh, P. W. (2008). Projected pain from noxious heat stimulation of an exposed peripheral nerve—A case report. *European Journal of Pain, 13,* 35–37.

Homer. (2006). *The Iliad* (S. Butler, Trans.; J. D. Pérezgonzález, Ed.). Raleigh, NC: Pergonomas. (Original work published c. 800 BCE in Greek)

Honeycutt, J. M. (2008). Imagined interaction theory. In. L. A. Baxter & D. O. Braithewaite (Eds.), *Engaging theory in interpersonal communication: Multiple perspectives* (pp. 77–87). Thousand Oaks, CA: Sage.

Honrubia, F. M., & Elliott, J. H. (1968). Efferent innervation of the retina. I. Morphologic study of the human retina. *Archives of Ophthalmology, 80,* 98–103.

Horselenberg, R., Merckelbach, H., Muris, P., Rassin, E., Sijsenaar, M., & Spaan, V. (2000). Imagining fictitious childhood events: The role of individual differences in imagination inflation. *Clinical Psychology & Psychotherapy, 7,* 128–137.

Horselenberg, R., Merckelbach, H., van Breukelen, G., & Wessel, I. (2004). Individual differences in the accuracy of autobiographical memory. *Clinical Psychology and Psychotherapy, 11,* 168–176.

Howell, T. J., & Bennett, P. C. (2011). Can dogs (Canis familiaris) use a mirror to solve a problem? *Journal of Veterinary Behavior: Clinical Applications and Research, 6,* 306–312.

Howie, P., Markham, R., & Kleitman, S. (2006). The development of imagery scales for children in three modalities. *Journal of Mental Imagery, 30*(1 & 2), 39–64.

Hughes, J. R. (1985). A review of the auditory system and its evoked potentials. *Journal of EEG Technology, 25,* 115–158.

Hume, D. (1896). *A treatise of human nature* (3 vols.). Oxford, UK: Clarendon Press. (Original work published 1739)

Hunt, D. M., Carvalho, L. S., Cowing, J. A., & Davies, W. L. (2009). Evolution and spectral tuning of visual pigments in birds and mammals. *Philosophical Transactions of the Royal Society: B. Biological Sciences, 364,* 2941–2955.

Huque, T., Cowart, B. J., Dankulich-Nagrudny, L., Pribitkin, E. A., Bayley, D. L., Spielman, et al. (2009). Sour ageusia in two individuals implicates ion channels of the ASIC and PKD families in human sour taste perception at the anterior tongue. *Plos One, 4,* e7347.

Hurvich, L. M., & Jameson, D. (1951). The binocular fusion of yellow in relation to color theories. *Science, 114,* 199–202.

Hutchison, W. D., Harfa, L., & Dostrovsky, J. O. (1996). Ventrolateral orbital cortex and periaqueductal gray stimulation-induced effects on on- and off-cells in the rostral ventromedial medulla in the rat. *Neuroscience, 70,* 391–407.

Hyatt, C. W., & Hopkins, W. D. (1994). Self-awareness in bonobos and chimpanzees: A comparative perspective. In S. T. Parker, R. W. Mitchell, & M. L. Boccia (Eds.), *Self-awareness in animals and humans: Developmental perspectives* (pp. 248–253). New York, NY: Cambridge University Press.

Hyman, I. E., Jr., & Billings, F. J. (1998). Individual differences and the creation of false childhood memories. *Memory, 6,* 1–20.

Ihara, M., & Kido, M. (1935). On the process of color mixtures (I). *Japanese Journal of Psychology, 10,* 725–745.

Ingvar, D. H. (1985). "Memory of the future": An essay on the temporal organization of conscious awareness. *Human Neurobiology, 4,* 127–136.

Irvine, D. R. F., & Webster, W. R. (1972). Arousal effects on cochlear potentials: Investigation of a two-factor hypothesis. *Brain Research, 39,* 109–119.

Ishihara, S. (1962). *The series of plates designed as a test for colour-blindness.* Tokyo, Japan: Kanehara Shuppan.

Ishii, T., Murakami, Y., & Balogh, K., Jr. (1967). Acetylcholinesterase activity in the efferent nerve fibers of the human inner ear. *Annals of Otology, Rhinology, and Laryngology, 76,* 69–82.

Iwaniuk, A. N., & Nelson, J. E. (2003). Developmental differences are correlated with relative brain size in birds: A comparative analysis. *Canadian Journal of Zoology, 81,* 1913–1928.

Izard, C. (1978). *Human emotions.* New York, NY: Plenum.

Jacoby, L. L., & Whitehouse, K. (1989). An illusion of memory: False recognition influence by unconscious perception. *Journal of Experimental Psychology: General, 118,* 126–135.

James, W. (1890). *The principles of psychology* (2 vols.). New York, NY: Henry Holt.

Jaynes, J. (1976). *The origin of consciousness in the breakdown of the bicameral mind.* Boston, MA: Houghton Mifflin.

Jerison, H. J. (1985). Animal intelligence as encephalization. *Philosophical Transactions of the Royal Society, B308,* 21–35.

Johnson, M. K. (1988). Reality monitoring: An experimental phenomenological approach. *Journal of Experimental Psychology: General, 117,* 390–394.

Johnson, M. K. (1991). Reflection, reality monitoring, and the self. In R. G. Kunzendorf (Ed.), *Mental imagery* (pp. 3–16). New York, NY: Plenum.

Jones, E. (1908). The precise diagnostic value of allochiria. *Brain: A Journal of Neurology, 30,* 490–532.

Jones, J. E., Antoniadis, E., Shettleworth, S. J., & Kamil, A. C. (2002). A comparative study of geometric rule learning by nutcrackers (*Nucifraga Columbiana*), pigeons (*Columba livia*), and jackdaws (*Corvus monedula*). *Journal of Comparative Psychology, 116,* 350–356.

Jordan, G., Deeb, S. S., Bosten, J. M., & Mollon, J. D. (2010). The dimensionality of color vision in carriers of anomalous trichromacy. *Journal of Vision, 10* (article 12), 1–19.

Jouvet, M. (1962). Recherches sur les structures nerveuses et les mécanismes responsables des différentes phases du sommeil physiologique. *Archives Italiennes de Biologie, 100,* 125–206.

Jouvet, M. (1967). Neurophysiology of the states of sleep. *Physiological Reviews, 47,* 117–177.

Julesz, B. (1971). *Foundations of cyclopean perception.* Chicago, IL: University of Chicago Press.

Kahan, T. L., & LaBerge, S. (1994). Lucid dreaming as metacognition: Implications for cognitive science. *Consciousness and Cognition, 3,* 246–264.

Kalil-Gaspar, P., Marcuzzo, S., Rigon, P., Molina, C. G., & Achaval, M. (2007). Capsaicin-induced avoidance behavior in the terrestrial Gastropoda Megalobulimus abbreviates: Evidence for TRPV-1 signaling and apioid modulation in response to chemical noxious stimuli. *Comparative Biochemistry and Physiology: Part A. Molecular & Integrative Physiology, 148,* 286–291.

Kamardin, N. N., Shalanki, Y., Rozha, K. S., & Nozdrachev, A. D. (2001). Studies of chemoreceptor perception in mollusks. *Neuroscience and Behavioral Physiology, 31,* 227–235.

Kambhampati, S. (1995). A phylogeny of cockroaches and related insects based on DNA sequence of mitochondrial ribosomal RNA genes. *Proceedings of the National Academy of Sciences, 92,* 2017–2020.

Kang, K., Pulver, S. R., Panzano, V. C., Chang, E. C., Griffith, L. C., Theobald, D. L.,_ & garrity, P. A. (2010). Analysis of *Drosophila* TRPA1 reveals an ancient origin for human chemical nociception. *Nature, 464,* 597–600.

Kantorowitz, D. A., & Cohen, B. D. (1977). Referent communication in chronic schizophrenia. *Journal of Abnormal Psychology, 86,* 1–9.

Kärtner, J., Keller, H., Chaudhary, N., & Yovsi, R. D. (2012). The development of mirror self-recognition in different sociocultural contexts. *Monographs of the Society for Research in Child Development, 77*(4), 1-87.

Kass-Simon, G., & Hufnagel, L. A. (1992). Suspected chemoreceptors in coelenterates and ctenophores. *Microscopy Research and Technique, 22,* 265–284.

Katayama, Y., Yamamoto, T., Kobayashi, K., Kasai, M., Oshima, H., & Fukaya, C. (2001). Motor cortex stimulation for post-stroke pain: Comparison of spinal cord and thalamic stimulation. *Stereotactic and Functional Neurosurgery, 77,* 183–186.

Katz, J. (1992). Psychophysical correlates of phantom limb experience. *Journal of Neurology, Neurosurgery, and Psychiatry, 55,* 811–821.

Katz, J. (1993). The reality of phantom limbs. *Motivation and Emotion, 17,* 147–179.

Katz, J. (2000). Individual differences in the consciousness of phantom limbs. In R. G. Kunzendorf & B. Wallace (Eds.), *Individual differences in conscious experience* (pp. 45–97). Amsterdam, The Netherlands: John Benjamins.

Kay, L. M., & Freeman, W. J. (1998). Bidirectional processing in the olfactory-limbic axis during olfactory behavior. *Behavioral Neuroscience, 112,* 541–553.

Kay, S. R., Fiszbein, A., & Opfer, L. A. (1987). The Positive and Negative Syndrome Scale (PANSS) for schizophrenia. *Schizophrenia Bulletin, 13,* 261–276.

Keil, T. A. (1997). Functional morphology of insect mechanoreceptors. *Microscopy Research and Technique, 39,* 506–531.

Keller, H., Kärtner, J., Borke, J., Yovsi, R., & Kleis, A. (2005). Parenting styles and the development of the categorical self: A longitudinal study on mirror self-recognition in Cameroonian Nso and German families. *International Journal of Behavioral Development, 29,* 496–504.

Keller, H., Yovsi, R., Borke, J., Kärtner, J., Jensen, H., & Papaligoura, Z. (2004). Developmental consequences of early parenting experiences: Self-recognition and self-regulation in three cultural communities. *Child Development, 75,* 1745–1760.

Kerr, D. I. B., & Hagbarth, K.-E. (1955). An investigation of olfactory centrifugal fiber system. *Journal of Neurophysiology, 18,* 362–374.

Kihlstrom, J. F., & Cantor, N. (1984). Mental representations of the self. In L. Berkowitz (Ed.), *Advances in experimental social psychology* (Vol. 17, pp. 1–47). Orlando, FL: Academic.

Kilcommons, A. M., & Morrison, A. P. (2005). Relationships between trauma and psychosis: An exploration of cognitive and dissociative factors. *Acta Psychiatrica Scandinavica, 112,* 351–359.

Kim, U., Wooding, S., Riaz, N., Jorde, L. B., & Drayna, D. (2006). Variation in the human TAS1R taste receptor genes. *Chemical Senses, 31,* 599–611.

Kim, U., Wooding, S., Ricci, D., Jorde, L. B., & Drayna, D. (2005). Worldwide haplotype diversity and coding sequence variation at human bitter taste receptor loci. *Human Mutation, 26,* 199–204.

Kingsley, H. L. (1932). An experimental study of "search." *American Journal of Psychology, 44,* 314–318.

Klinger, E. (1992). Motivation and imagination. *Psychologische Beitrage, 34,* 127–142.

Kluft, R. P. (1987). First-rank symptoms as a diagnostic clue to Multiple Personality Disorder. *American Journal of Psychiatry, 144,* 293–298.

Koestenbaum, P. (1964–1965). The vitality of death. *Journal of Existentialism, 5,* 139–166.

Komatsu, H. (1998). Mechanisms of central color vision. *Current Opinion in Neurobiology, 8,* 503–508.

Kosslyn, S. M. (1994). *Image and brain*. Cambridge, MA: MIT Press.

Kosslyn, S. M., Brunn, J., Cave, K., & Wallach, R. (1984). Individual differences in mental imagery ability: A componential analysis. *Cognition, 18,* 195–243.

Kovács, I., Papathomas, T. V., Yang, M., & Fehér, A. (1996). When the brain changes its mind: Interocular grouping during binocular rivalry. *Proceedings of the National Academy of Sciences of the United States of America, 93,* 15505–15511.

Kozmik, Z. (2008). The role of Pax genes in eye evolution. *Brain Research Bulletin, 75,* 335–339.

Külpe, O. (1895). *Outlines of psychology* (E. B. Titchener, Trans.). London, UK: Sonnenschein. (Original work published 1893 under the German title *Grundriss der Psychologie*)

Kunze, W. A., Shafton, A. D., Kemm, R. E., & McKenzie, J. S. (1991). Effect of stimulating the nucleus of the horizontal limb of the diagonal band on single unit activity in the olfactory bulb. *Neuroscience, 40,* 21–27.

Kunzendorf, R. G. (1980). Imagery and consciousness: A scientific analysis of the mind-body problem. *Dissertation Abstract International: Section B. Science and Engineering, 40,* 3448–3449.

Kunzendorf, R. G. (1982). Mental images, appreciation of grammatical patterns, and creativity. *Journal of Mental Imagery, 6,* 183–202.

Kunzendorf, R. G. (1984). Centrifugal effects of eidetic imaging on flash electroretinograms and autonomic responses. *Journal of Mental Imagery, 8*(4), 67–76.

Kunzendorf, R. G. (1984–1985). Subconscious percepts as "unmonitored" percepts. *Imagination, Cognition and Personality, 4,* 367–375.

Kunzendorf, R. G. (1985–1986a). Hypnotic hallucinations as "unmonitored" images. *Imagination, Cognition and Personality, 5,* 255–270.

Kunzendorf, R. G. (1985–1986b). Repressed fear of inexistence and its hypnotic recovery in religious subjects. *Omega: Journal of Death and Dying, 16,* 23–33.

Kunzendorf, R. G. (1987–1988). Self-consciousness as the monitoring of cognitive states. *Imagination, Cognition and Personality, 7,* 3–22.

Kunzendorf, R. G. (1989). Afterimages of eidetic images: A developmental study. *Journal of Mental Imagery, 13*(1), 55–62.

Kunzendorf, R. G. (1989–1990). Posthypnotic amnesia: Dissociation of self-concept or self-consciousness? *Imagination, Cognition and Personality, 9,* 321–334.

Kunzendorf, R. G. (1990). Mind-brain identity theory: A materialistic foundation for the psychophysiology of mental imagery. In R. G. Kunzendorf & A. A. Sheikh (Eds.), *The psychophysiology of mental imagery* (pp. 9–36). Amityville, NY: Baywood.

Kunzendorf, R. G. (1990–1991). Consciousness in contemporary science. (A. Marcel & E. Bisiach, Eds.). *Imagination, Cognition and Personality, 10,* 104–107.

Kunzendorf, R. G. (1992–1993). Effect of image vividness on reality monitoring. *Imagination, Cognition and Personality, 12,* 197–205.

Kunzendorf, R. G. (2000). Individual differences in self-conscious source monitoring: Theoretical, experimental, and clinical considerations. In R. G. Kunzendorf & B. Wallace (Eds.), *Individual differences in conscious experience* (pp. 375–390). Amsterdam, The Netherlands: John Benjamins.

Kunzendorf, R. G. (2006). Universal repression from consciousness *versus* abnormal dissociation from self-consciousness. *Behavioral & Brain Sciences, 29,* 523–524.

Kunzendorf, R. G. (2007a). Confronting death through mental and artistic imagery. In A. A. Sheikh & K. S. Sheikh (Eds.), *Healing with death imagery* (pp. 47–65). Amityville, NY: Baywood.

Kunzendorf, R. G. (2007b). Is binocular fusion of "cortical yellow" an illusion, contingent upon abstraction of coherent sensory information from the two eyes? *Perceptual and Motor Skills, 104,* 298–306.

Kunzendorf, R. G. (2007c). Symbolic images in dreams and daydreams. In P. McNamara & D. Barrett (Eds.), *The new science of dreaming* (Vol. 3, pp. 155–170). Westport, CT: Greenwood.

Kunzendorf, R. G. (2009). Binocular perception of an abstract multicolored display through one red-filtered eye and one green-filtered eye. *Perceptual and Motor Skills, 109,* 707–717.

Kunzendorf, R. G. (2010). The hypnotic deactivation of self-conscious source monitoring. In D. Barrett (Ed.), *Hypnosis and hypnotherapy* (Vol. 1, pp. 1–14). Santa Barbara, CA: ABC-CLIO.

Kunzendorf, R. G. (2014). Phenomenal yellow from rotated red and green: Retinal qualia versus emergent cortical qualia. *Psychology of Consciousness, 1,* 320–328.

Kunzendorf, R. G., & Boisvert, P. (1996). Presence vs. absence of a "hidden observer" during total deafness: The hypnotic illusion of subconsciousness vs. the imaginal attenuation of brainstem evoked potentials. In R. G. Kunzendorf, N. P. Spanos, & B. Wallace (Eds.), *Hypnosis and imagination* (pp. 223–234). Amityville, NY: Baywood.

Kunzendorf, R. G., & Buker, F. (2007–2008). Does existential meaning require hope, *or* is interest enough? *Imagination, Cognition and Personality, 27,* 233–243.

Kunzendorf, R. G., & Buker, F. (2008–2009). Should visual images be defined as depictive neural patterns, *or* as conscious sensations constructed from "imageless" visual thoughts? *Imagination, Cognition and Personality, 28,* 5–35.

Kunzendorf, R. G., & Butler, W. (1992). Apperception revisited: "Subliminal" monocular perception during the apperception of fused random-dot stereograms. *Consciousness and Cognition, 1,* 63–76.

Kunzendorf, R. G., Butler, W., & Pearson, B. (1988). Are monocular arrays discriminable from binocular arrays? *Perceptual and Motor Skills, 66,* 531–534.

Kunzendorf, R. G., Connors, J., Arrecis, C., Farrington, J., & Carter, S. (2008–2009). Do psychologically autonomous individuals behave as if they have free will? *Imagination, Cognition and Personality, 28,* 269–281.

Kunzendorf, R. G., Crosson, M., Zalaket, A., White, J., & Enik, R. (1998–1999). Normal dimensions of multiple personality without amnesia. *Imagination, Cognition and Personality, 18,* 205–221.

Kunzendorf, R. G., Deignan, M., Galva, M., Latorre, K., & Masotta, E. (2005-2006). The psychological boundaries delineating truth and falsehood. *Imagination, Cognition and Personality, 25,* 283–297.

Kunzendorf, R. G., DeJesus, N., Chicos, N., & Avalos, H. (2000-2001). Resolving existential sentiments with music: Evidence for a "mental chemistry" of emotions. *Imagination, Cognition and Personality, 20,* 59–69.

Kenzendord, R. G., Dohery, K. R., Jr., Visconti, T. P., Giacalone, C. M., & Vangapalli, R. R. (2015–2016). Existential authenticily: Exploratory factor analyses. *Imagination, Cognition, and Personality, 35,* in press.

Kunzendorf, R. G., Dwyer, N., Foran, M., Pagan, A., Giuseppe, A., & Milligan, B. (2013–2014). Heterarchical versus hierarchical modes of imageless thinking. *Imagination, Cognition and Personality, 33*, 403–420.

Kunzendorf, R. G., Francis, L., Ward, J., Cohen, R., Cutler, J., Walsh, J., et al. (1996–1997). Effect of negative imaging on heart rate and blood pressures, as a function of image vividness and image "realness." *Imagination, Cognition and Personality, 16,* 139–159.

Kunzendorf, R. G., & Hall, S. (2001). Electroretinographic after-effects of visual imaging: Individual differences in imagery vividness and reality testing. *Journal of Mental Imagery, 25*(2), 79–92.

Kunzendorf, R. G., Hartmann, E., Thomas, L., & Berensen, L. (1999–2000). Emotionally directing visual sensations: I. Generating images that contextualize emotion and become "symbolic." *Imagination, Cognition and Personality, 19,* 269–278.

Kunzendorf, R. G., Hulihan, D., Simpson, W., Pritykina, N., & Williams, K. (1997-1998). Is absorption a diathesis for dissociation in sexually and physically abused patients? *Imagination, Cognition and Personality, 17,* 277–282.

Kunzendorf, R. G., Jesses, M., Michaels, A., Ciazzo-Fluellen, G., & Butler, W. (1991). Imagination and perceptual development: Effects of auditory imaging on the brainstem evoked potentials of children, adult musicians and other adults. In R. G. Kunzendorf (Ed.), *Mental imagery* (pp. 159–166). New York, NY: Plenum.

Kunzendorf, R. G., Justice, M., & Capone, D. (1997). Conscious images as "centrally excited sensations": A developmental study of imaginal influences on the ERG. *Journal of Mental Imagery, 21*(1 & 2), 155–166.

Kunzendorf, R. G., & Karpen, J. (1996–1997). Dissociative experiences and reality-testing deficits in college students. *Imagination, Cognition and Personality, 16,* 227–238.

Kunzendorf, R. G., Leszkiewicz, J., Hamill, K., McAleer, S., Geoffroy, S., Ciampaglia, A., Pereira, D., & Brito, C. (2006–2007). Dreaming and daydreaming about dreadful possibilities: Primal fears versus existential fears. *Imagination, Cognition and Personality, 26,* 249–257.

Kunzendorf, R. G., Lyman, S. S., Sousa, B., & Hilly, E. (2012–2013). "Imageless" spatial and temporal rules can be tested and refined by constructing vivid visual and auditory images. *Imagination, Cognition and Personality, 32*, 115–150.

Kunzendorf, R. G., & McGlinchey-Berroth, R. (1997–1998). The return of "the subliminal." *Imagination, Cognition and Personality, 17,* 31–43.

Kunzendorf, R. G., & McLaughlin, S. (1988–1989). Depression: A failure to suppress the self-conscious "monitoring" of dismal cognitions. *Imagination, Cognition and Personality, 8,* 3–17.

Kunzendorf, R. G., McLaughlin-Beltz, S., & Tymowicz, G. (1991). Self-awareness in autistic subjects and deeply hypnotized subjects: Dissociation of self-concept versus self-consciousness. *Imagination, Cognition and Personality, 11,* 129–141.

Kunzendorf, R. G., & Moran, C. (1993–1994). Repression: Active censorship of stressful memories vs. source amnesia for self-consciously dissociated memories. *Imagination, Cognition and Personality, 13,* 291–302.

Kunzendorf, R. G., Moran, C., & Gray, R. (1995–1996). Personality traits and reality-testing abilities, controlling for vividness of imagery. *Imagination, Cognition and Personality, 15,* 113–131.

Kunzendorf, R. G., & Reynolds, K. (2004-2005). On the cognitive function of visual images and the development of individual differences. *Imagination, Cognition and Personality, 24,* 245–257.

Kunzendorf, R. G., Thompson, D., & Butler, W. (1995–1996). Percepts considered as "bundles of sensations": Confusion of percepts with afterimages. *Imagination, Cognition and Personality, 15*, 309–318.

Kunzendorf, R. G., Treantafel, N., Taing, B., Flete, A., Savoie, S., Agersea, S., & Williams, R. (2006–2007). The sense of self in lucid dreams: "Self as subject" vs. "self as agent" vs. "self as object." *Imagination, Cognition and Personality, 26,* 303–324.

Kunzendorf, R. G., Young, K., Beecy, T., & Beals, K. (2000). Is visual thinking "imageless thought"? *Perceptual and Motor Skills, 91,* 981–982.

Kupers, R., Fumal, A., de Noordhout, A. M., Gjedde, A., Schoenen, J., & Ptito, M. (2006). Transcranial magnetic stimulation of the visual cortex induces somatotopically organized qualia in blind subjects. *Proceedings of the National Academy of Sciences, 103,* 13256–13260.

LaBerge, S. (1985). *Lucid dreaming.* New York, NY: Ballantine.

LaBerge, S., & DeGracia, D. J. (2000). Varieties of lucid dreaming experience. In R. G. Kunzendorf & B. Wallace (Eds.), *Individual differences in conscious experience* (pp. 269–307). Amsterdam, The Netherlands: John Benjamins.

Laeng, B., & Teodorescu, D.-S. (2002). Eye scanpaths during visual imagery reenact those of perception of the same visual scene. *Cognitive Science, 26,* 207–231.

Larhammar, D., Nordström, K., & Larsson, T. A. (2009). Evolution of rod and cone phototransduction genes. *Philosophical Transactions of the Royal Society: B. Biological Sciences, 364,* 2867–2880.

Lee, H., Voss, M. W., Prakash, R. S., Boot, W. R., Vo, L. T. K., Basak, C., et al. (2012). Videogame training strategy-induced change in brain function during a complex visuomotor task. *Behavioural Brain Research, 232,* 348–357.

Lee, H. W., Hong, S. B., Seo, D. W., Tae, W. S., & Hong, S. C. (2000). Mapping of functional organization in human visual cortex: Electrical cortical stimulation. *Neurology, 54,* 849–854.

Lefebvre, L., Reader, S. M., & Sol, D. (2004). Brains, innovations and evolution in birds and primates. *Brain, Behavior, and Evolution, 63,* 233–246.

Leibniz, G. W. (1896). *New essays concerning human understanding* (A. G. Langley, Trans.). New York, NY: Macmillan. (Original work published 1765)

Leonard, G., & Lindauer, M. S. (1973). Aesthetic participation and imagery arousal. *Perceptual and Motor Skills, 36,* 977–978.

Leslie, A. M. (1987). Pretense and representation: The origins of "theory of mind." *Psychological Review, 94,* 412–426.

Levenson, R. W. (1994). The search for autonomic specificity. In P. Ekman & R. J. Davidson (Eds.), *The nature of emotion: Fundamental questions* (pp. 252–257). New York, NY: Oxford University Press.

Lewis, M., & Ramsay, D. (2004). Development of self-recognition, personal pronoun use, and pretend play during the 2nd year. *Child Development, 75,* 1821–1831.

Li, H., Pakstis, A. J., Kidd, J. R., & Kidd, K. K. (2011). Selection on the human bitter taste gene, TAS2R16, in Eurasian populations. *Human Biology, 83,* 363–377.

Libet, B. (1973). Electrical stimulation of cortex in human subjects and conscious sensory aspects. In A. Iggo (Ed.), *Handbook of sensory physiology* (Vol. II, pp. 743–790). Berlin, Germany: Springer-Verlag.

Libet, B., Wright, E. W., Feinstein, B., & Pearl, D. K. (1979). Subjective referral of the timing for a conscious sensory experience: A functional role for the somato-sensory specific projection system in man. *Brain: A Journal of Neurology, 102,* 193–224.

Lim, H. H., & Anderson, D. J. (2007). Antidromic activation reveals tonotopically organized projections from primary auditory cortex to the central nucleus of the infer colliculus in guinea pig. *Journal of Neurophysiology, 97,* 1413–1427.

Lindauer, M. S. (1977). Imagery from the point of view of psychological aesthetics, the arts, and creativity. *Journal of Mental Imagery, 2,* 343–362.

Logie, R. H., Pernet, C. R., Buonocore, A., & Della Sala, S. (2011). Low and high imagers activate networks differentially in mental rotation. *Neuropsychologia, 49,* 3071–3077.

Lorenz, C., & Neisser, U. (1985). Factors of imagery and event recall. *Memory and Cognition, 13,* 494–500.

Lörincz, M. L., Oláh, M., & Juhász, G. (2008). Functional consequences of retinopetal fibers originating in the dorsal raphe nucleus. *International Journal of Neuroscience, 118,* 1374–1383.

Low, P. S., Shank, S. S., Sejnowski, T. J., & Margoliash, D. (2008). Mammalian-like features of sleep structure in zebra finches. *Proceedings of the National Academy of Sciences, 105,* 9081–8086.

Lozano, A. M., Hutchison, W. E., Tasker, R. R., Lang, A. E., Junn, F., & Dostrovsky, J. O. (1998). Microelectrode recordings define the ventral posteromedial pallidotomy target. *Stereotactic and Functional Neurosurgery, 71,* 153–163.

Lukas, J. H. (1980). Human auditory attention: The olivocochlear bundle may function as a peripheral filter. *Psychophysiology, 17,* 444–452.

Lukas, J. H. (1981). The role of efferent inhibition in human auditory attention: An examination of auditory brainstem potentials. *International Journal of Neuroscience, 12,* 137–145.

Luu, B. L., Day, B. L., Cole, J. D., & Fitzpatrick, R. C. (2011). The fusimotor and reafferent origin of the sense of force and weight. *Journal of Physiology, 589,* 3135–3147.

Lyamin, O. I., Shpak, O. V., Nazarenko, E. A., & Mukhametov, L. M. (2002). Muscle jerks during behavioral sleep in a beluga whale. *Physiology & Behavior, 76,* 265–270.

Lyn, H., Greenfield, P., & Savage-Rumbaugh, S. (2006). The development of representational play in chimpanzees and bonobos: Evolutionary implications, pretense, and the role of interspecies communication. *Cognitive Development, 21,* 199–213.

Lynn, S. J., Lilienfeld, S. O., Merckelbach, H., Giesbrecht, T., & van der Kloet, D. (2012). Dissociation and dissociative disorders: Challenging conventional wisdom. *Current Directions in Psychological Science, 21,* 48–53.

Ma, M., & Luo, M. (2012). Optogenetic activation of basal forebrain cholinergic neurons modulates neuronal excitability and sensory responses in the main olfactory bulb. *Journal of Neuroscience, 32,* 10105–10116.

Maaswinkel, H., & Li, L. (2003). Olfactory input increases visual sensitivity in zebrafish: A possible function for the terminal nerve and dopaminergic interplexiform cells. *Journal of Experimental Biology, 206,* 2201–2209.

Macphail, E. M. (1998). *The evolution of consciousness.* Oxford, UK: Oxford University Press.

Mandes, E. (1985). Interposition and size constancy: A developmental study. *Perceptual and Motor Skills, 61,* 196–198.

Mangun, G. R., Hansen, J. C., & Hillyard, S. A. (1986). Electroretinograms reveal no evidence for centrifugal modulation of retinal inputs during selective attention in man. *Psychophysiology, 23,* 156–165.

Manley, G. A. (2000). Cochlear mechanisms from a phylogenetic viewpoint. *Proceedings of the National Academy of Sciences, 97,* 11736–11743.

Manouélian, Y. (1898). Contribution à l'étude du bulbe olfactif: Hypothese des nervi-nerorum. *Comptes Rendus des Séances de la Société de Biologie et des ses Filiales, 10e S*(5), 194–195.

Marino, L., Reiss, D., & Gallup, G. G., Jr. (1994). Mirror self-recognition in bottlenose dolphins: Implications for comparative investigation in highly dissimilar species. In S. T. Parker, R. W. Mitchell, & M. L. Boccia (Eds.), *Self-awareness in animals and humans: Developmental perspectives* (pp. 380–391). New York, NY: Cambridge University Press.

Markham, R., & Hynes, L. (1993). The effect of vividness of imagery on reality monitoring. *Journal of Mental Imagery, 177*(3 & 4), 159–170.

Marks, D. F. (1973). Visual imagery differences in the recall of pictures. *British Journal of Psychology, 64,* 17–24.

Marten, K., & Psarakos, S. (1994). Evidence of self-awareness in the bottlenose dolphin (Tursiops truncates). In S. T. Parker, R. W. Mitchell, & M. L. Boccia (Eds.), *Self-awareness in animals and humans: Developmental perspectives* (pp. 361–379). New York, NY: Cambridge University Press.

Matsuyama, M. (1967). Existence of centrifugal nerve fiber in the retina. *Jahresbericht Kurashiki Zentral Hospital, 36,* 1–23.

Maxwell, J. C. (1855). Experiments on colour as perceived by the eye. *Transactions of the Royal Society of Edinburgh, 21*, 274–299.

McBride, C. S., & Arguello, J. R. (2007). Five Drosophila genomes reveal nonneutral evolution and the signature of host specialization in the chemoreceptor superfamily. *Genetics, 177,* 1395–1416.

McCune, L., & Agayoff, J. (2002). Pretending as representation: A developmental and comparative review. In R. W. Mitchell (Ed.), *Pretending and imagination in animals and children* (pp. 43–55). Cambridge, UK: Cambridge University Press.

McDougall, W. (1911). *Body and mind: A history and a defense of animism.* London, UK: Methuen.

McElroy, S. L., Strakowski, S. M., West, S. A., Keck, P. E., Jr., & McConville, B. J. (1997). Phenomenology of adolescent and adult mania in hospitalized patients with bipolar disorder. *American Journal of Psychiatry, 154,* 44–49.

McGlone, F., & Reilly, D. (2010). The cutaneous sensory system. *Neuroscience and Biobehavioral Reviews, 34,* 148–159.

McGuffin, P., Reveley, A., & Holland, A. (1982). Identical triplets: Non-identical psychosis? *British Journal of Psychiatry, 140,* 1–6.

McKelvie, S. J. (1995). The VVIQ as a psychometric test of individual differences in visual imagery vividness: A critical quantitative review and plea for direction. *Journal of Mental Imagery, 19*(3 & 4), 1–106, 192–252.

McKelvie, S. J., & Rohrberg, M. M. (1978). Individual differences in reported visual imagery and cognitive performance. *Perceptual and Motor Skills, 46,* 451–458.

McKemy, D. D. (2007). Temperature sensing across species. *Pflügers Archiv: European Journal of Physiology, 454,* 777–791.

McMahon, C. E. (1973). Images as motives and motivators: A historical perspective. *American Journal of Psychology, 86,* 465–490.

McMahon, C. E. (1974). Voluntary control of "involuntary" functions: The approach of the Stoics. *Psychophysiology, 11,* 710–714.

McMahon, C. E. (1976). The role of imagination in the disease process: Pre-Cartesian history. *Psychological Medicine, 6,* 179–184.

McNamara, P. (2004). *An evolutionary psychology of sleep and dreams.* Westport, CT: Praeger.

Medina, F. S., Taylor, A. H., Hunt, G. R., & Gray, R. D. (2011). New Caledonian crows' responses to mirrors. *Animal Behaviour, 82,* 981–993.

Menninger, K., Ellenberger, H., Pruyser, P., & Mayman, M. (1958). The unitary concept of mental illness. *Bulletin of the Menninger Clinic, 22,* 1–12.

Merbs, S. L., & Nathans, J. (1992a). Absorption spectra of human cone pigments. *Nature, 356,* 433–435.

Merbs, S. L., & Nathans, J. (1992b). Photobleaching difference absorption spectra of human cone pigments: Quantitative analysis and comparison to other methods. *Photochemistry and Photobiology, 56,* 869–881.

Merker, B. (2007). Consciousness without a cerebral cortex: A challenge for neuroscience and medicine. *Behavioral and Brain Sciences, 30,* 63–134.

Meyer, M. F. (1922). *Psychology of the other one*. Columbus, MO: Missouri Books.

Miles, H. L. W. (1994). Me Chantek: The development of self-awareness in a signing orangutan. In S. T. Parker, R. W. Mitchell, & M. L. Boccia (Eds.), *Self-awareness in animals and humans: Developmental perspectives* (pp. 254–272). New York, NY: Cambridge University Press.

Millan, M. J. (1999). The induction of pain: An integrative review. *Progress in Neurobiology, 57,* 1–164.

Millan, M. J. (2002). Descending control of pain. *Progress in Neurobiology, 66,* 355–474.

Miller, A. I. (1986). *Imagery in scientific thought*. Cambridge, MA: MIT Press.

Millon, T. (1994). *Millon Clinical Multiaxial Inventory-III manual*. Minneapolis, MN: National Computer Systems.

Milton, J. (1962). *Paradise lost: A poem in twelve books* (M. Y. Hughes, Ed.). New York, NY: Odyssey Press. (Original work published 1674)

Mintz, S., & Alpert, M. (1972). Imagery vividness, reality testing, and schizophrenic hallucinations. *Journal of Abnormal Psychology, 79,* 310–316.

Mitchell, R. W. (2013). The comparative study of imagination. In M. Taylor (Ed.), *Oxford handbook of the development of imagination* (pp. 468–485). New York, NY: Oxford University Press.

Mogensen, J., & Divac, I. (1982). The prefrontal "cortex" in the pigeon: Behavioral evidence. *Brain, Behavior and Evolution, 21,* 60–66.

Mori, F., & Ronchi, L. (1960). Unusual factors influencing the electroretinographic intensity function. *Atti della Fondazione Giorgo Ronchi, 15,* 503–510.

Morrison, A. P., & Haddock, G. (1997). Cognitive factors in source monitoring and auditory hallucinations. *Psychological Medicine, 27,* 669–679.

Morrison, R. G., & Wallace, B. (2001). Imagery vividness, creativity and the visual arts. *Journal of Mental Imagery, 25*(3 & 4), 135–152.

Moskowitz, A. (2004). Dissociation and violence: A review of the literature. *Trauma, Violence, & Abuse, 5,* 21–46.

Moskowitz, A., & Corstens, D. (2007). Auditory hallucinations: Psychotic symptom or dissociative experience? *Journal of Psychological Trauma, 6,* 35–63.

Motokawa, K., & Ebe, M. (1954). Antidromic stimulation of optic nerve and photosensitivity of cat retina. *Journal of Neurophysiology, 17,* 364–374.

Mulders, W. H. A. M., & Robertson, D. (2000). Effects on cochlear responses of activation of descending pathway from the inferior colliculus. *Hearing Research, 149,* 11–23.

Nafe, J. P. (1927). Dermal sensitivity with special reference to the qualities of tickle and itch. *Pedagogical Seminary and Journal of Genetic Psychology, 34,* 14–27.

Nagasako, E. M., Oaklander, A. L., & Dworkin, R. H. (2003). Congenital insensitivity to pain: An update. *Pain, 101,* 213–219.

Nagel, T. (1974). What is it like to be a bat? *Philosophical Review, 83,* 435–350.

Nagel, T. (1993). What is the mind-body problem? In *Experimental and theoretical studies of consciousness* (*Ciba Foundation Symposium, 174,* pp. 1–13). Chichester, UK: John Wiley.

Nakamura, H., Kojima, S., Kobayashi, S., Ito, I., Fujito, Y., Suzuki, H., & Ito, E. (1999). Physiological characterization of lip and tentacle nerves in Lymnaea stagnalis. *Neuroscience Research, 33,* 291–298.

National Institute of Mental Health. (1966). *Current research on sleep and dreams.* Bethesda, MD: National Institutes of Health, U.S. Department of Health, Education, and Welfare. (Public Health Service Publication No. 1389)

Natsoulas, T. (1989-1990). The self of all other selves: Part I. *Imagination, Cognition and Personality, 9,* 335–354.

Natsoulas, T. (2000-2001). The stream of consciousness: XXI. Blindsight and states of consciousness. *Imagination, Cognition and Personality, 20,* 71–95.

Ndetei, D. M., & Singh, A. (1983). Hallucinations in Kenyan schizophrenic patients. *Acta Psychiatrica Scandinavica, 67,* 144–147.

Neary, J. T., Crow, T., & Alkon, D. L. (1981). Change in a specific phosphoprotein band following associative learning in Hermissenda. *Nature, 293,* 658–660.

Neisser, U. (1976). *Cognition and reality: Principles and implications of cognitive psychology.* New York, NY: W. H. Freeman.

Nelson, R. E., & Craighead, W. (1977). Selective recall of positive and negative feedback, self-control, and depression. *Journal of Abnormal Psychology, 86,* 379–388.

Nicholls, J. G., & Baylor, D. A. (1968). Specific modalities and receptive fields of sensory neurons in CNS of the leech. *Journal of Neurophysiology, 31,* 740–756.

Nicol, S. C., Andersen, N. A., Phillips, N. H., & Berger, R. J. (2000). The echidna manifests typical characteristics of rapid eye movement sleep. *Neuroscience Letters, 283,* 49–52.

Niedźwieńska, A. (2000–2001). Imagination and source monitoring accuracy. *Imagination, Cognition and Personality, 20,* 21–31.

Nielsen, M., & Dissanayake, C. (2004). Pretend play, mirror self-recognition and imitation: A longitudinal investigation through the second year. *Infant Behavior & Development, 27,* 342–365.

Nienow, T. M., & Docherty, N. M. (2004). Internal source monitoring and thought disorder in schizophrenia. *Journal of Nervous and Mental Disease, 192,* 696–700.

Nomura, Y., & Schuknecht, H. F. (1965). The efferent fibers in the cochlea. *Annals of Otology, Rhinology, and Laryngology, 74,* 289–302.

Nordström, K., Wallén, R., Seymour, J., & Nilsson, D. (2003). A simple visual system without neurons in jellyfish larvae. *Proceedings of the Royal Society: B. Biological Sciences, 270,* 2349–2354.

Ogden, T. E., & Brown, K. T. (1964). Intraretinal responses of the cynamolgus monkey to electrical stimulation of the optic nerve and retina. *Journal of Neurophysiology, 27,* 682–705.

Ohlrogge, M., Doucet, J. R., & Ryugo, D. K. (2001). Projections of the pontine nuclei to the cochlear nucleus in rats. *Journal of Comparative Neurology, 436,* 290–303.

Okun, M. S., Mann, G., Foote, K. D., Shapira, N. A., Bowers, D., Springer, U., et al. (2007). Deep brain stimulation in the internal capsule and nucleus accumbens region: Responses observed during active and sham programming. *Journal of Neurology, Neurosurgery & Psychiatry, 78,* 310–314.

Olson, R. K. (1975). Children's sensitivity to pictorial depth information. *Perception & Psychophysics, 17,* 59–64.

Ono, H., & Barbeito, R. (1985). Utrocular discrimination is not sufficient for utrocular identification. *Vision Research, 25,* 289–299.

Osorio, D., & Vorobyev, M. (2008). A review of the evolution of animal colour vision and visual communication signals. *Vision Research, 48,* 2042–2051.

Paddock, J. R., Noel, M., Terranova, S., Eber, H. W., Manning, C., & Loftus, E. F. (1999). Imagination inflation and the perils of guided visualization. *Journal of Psychology: Interdisciplinary and Applied, 133,* 581–595.

Palacious, A. G., & Goldsmith, T. H. (1993). Photocurrents in retinal rods of pigeons (*Columba Livia*): Kinetics and spectral sensitivity. *Journal of Physiology, 471,* 817–829.

Parker, A. (2003). *In the blink of an eye.* New York, NY: Perseus.

Parker, S. T. (1994). Incipient mirror self-recognition in zoo gorillas and chimpanzees. In S. T. Parker, R. W. Mitchell, & M. L. Boccia (Eds.), *Self-awareness in animals and humans: Developmental perspectives* (pp. 301–307). New York, NY: Cambridge University Press.

Parrott, C. A. (1986). Visual imagery training: Stimulating utilization of imaginal processes. *Journal of Mental Imagery, 10*(1), 47–64.

Pastor, J., Soria, B., & Belmonte, C. (1996). Properties of nociceptive neurons of leech segmental ganglion. *Journal of Neurophysiology, 75,* 2268–2279.

Patterson, F. G. P., & Cohn, R. H. (1994). Self-recognition and self-awareness in lowland gorillas. In S. T. Parker, R. W. Mitchell, & M. L. Boccia (Eds.), *Self-awareness in animals and humans: Developmental perspectives* (pp. 273–290). New York, NY: Cambridge University Press.

Patzke, N., Manns, M., & Güntürkün, O. (2011). Telencephalic organization of the olfactory system in homing pigeons (*Columba livia*). *Neuroscience, 194,* 53–61.

Pavlov, I. P. (1927). *Conditioned reflexes: An investigation of the physiological activity of the cerebral cortex* (G. V. Anrep, Trans.). Oxford, UK: Oxford University Press.

Peachey, N. S., Alexander, K. R., Fishman, G. A., & Derlacki, D. J. (1989). Properties of the human cone system electroretinogram during light adaptation. *Applied Optics, 28,* 1145–1150.

Peachey, N. S., Arakawa, K., Alexander, K. R., & Marchese, A. L. (1992). Rapid and slow changes in the human cone electroretinogram during light and dark adaptation. *Vision Research, 32,* 2049–2053.

Penfield, W., & Rasmussen, T. (1955). *The cerebral cortex of man.* New York, NY: Macmillan.

Pepper, S. C. (1960). A neural-identity theory of mind. In S. Hook (Ed.), *Dimensions of mind* (pp. 45–61). London, UK: Collier Macmillan.

Pepperberg, I. M., Garcia, S. E., Jackson, E. C., & Marconi, S. (1995). Mirror use by African grey parrots (*Psittacus erithacus*). *Journal of Comparative Psychology, 109,* 182–195.

Pérez-Fabello, M. J., & Campos, A. (2007). Influence of training in artistic skills on mental imaging capacity. *Creativity Research Journal, 19,* 227–232.

Perky, C. W. (1910). An experimental study of imagination. *American Journal of Psychology, 21,* 422–452.

Perona-Garcelán, S., García-Montes, J. M., Ductor-Recuerda, M. J., Vallina-Fernández, O., Cuevas-Yust, C., Pérez-Álvarez, M., Salas-Azcona, R., & Gómez, M. T. (2012). Relationship of megacognition, absorption, and depersonalization in patients with auditory hallucinations. *British Journal of Clinical Psychology, 51,* 100–118.

Perrot, X., Ryvlin, P., Isnard, J., Guénot, M., Catenoix, H., Fischer, C., Mauguiére, F., & Collet, L. (2006). Evidence for corticofugal modulation of peripheral auditory activity in humans. *Cerebral Cortex, 16,* 941–948.

Pescetto, G., & Dettore, D. (1981). Fototattismo negative e condizionamento nellaplanaria Dugesia dorotocephala [Negative phototaxis and conditioning in the planarian Dugesia dorotocephala]. *Rivista di Neurobiologia, 10,* 287–295.

Piaget, J. (1932). *The moral judgment of the child.* (M. Gabain, Trans.). New York, NY: Harcourt, Brace.

Piaget, J. (1970) *Genetic epistemology* (E. Duckworth, Trans.). New York, NY: Columbia University Press.

Piaget, J. (1972). Intellectual evolution from adolescence to adulthood. *Human Development, 15,* 1–12.

Piaget, J., & Inhelder, B. (1947). Diagnosis of mental operations and theory of the intelligence. *American Journal of Mental Deficiency, 51,* 401–406.

Piaget, J., & Inhelder, B. (1971). *Mental imagery in the child: A study of the development of imaginal representation.* New York, NY: Basic.

Picton, T. W., Hillyard, S. A., Krausz, H. I., & Galambos, R. (1974). Human auditory evoked potentials. I.: Evaluation of components. *Electroencephalography and Clinical Neurophysiology, 36,* 179–190.

Pierce, J. (2012). *The last walk: Reflections on our pets at the end of their lives.* Chicago, IL: University of Chicago Press.

Pietrini, P., Furey, M. L., Ricciardi, E., Gobbini, M. I., Wu, W. H., Cohen, L., Guazzelli, M., & Haxby, J. V. (2004). Beyond sensory images: Object-based representation in the human ventral pathway. *Proceedings of the National Academy of Sciences, 101,* 5658–5663.

Pinel, J. P. J. (1997). *Biopsychology* (3rd ed.). Boston, MA: Allyn & Bacon.

Platt, C. J. (1973). Central control of postural orientation in flatfish. *Dissertation Abstracts International, 33(10–B)*, 4686.

Plotnik, J. M., de Waal, F. B. M., & Reiss, D. (2006). Self-recognition in an Asian elephant. *Proceedings of the National Academy of Sciences, 103,* 17053–17057.

Pockett, S. (2004). Does consciousness cause behavior? *Journal of Consciousness Studies, 11,* 23–40.

Poltrock, S. E., & Brown, P. (1984). Individual differences in visual imagery and spatial ability. *Intelligence, 8,* 93–138.

Posada, S., & Colell, M. (2007). Another gorilla (*Gorilla gorilla gorilla*) recognizes himself in a mirror. *American Journal of Primatology, 69,* 576–583.

Powell, M. (2005, May 23–29). A doubting rationalist: "Intelligent design" proponent Phillip Johnson, and how he came to be. *The Washington Post National Weekly Edition*, 11–12.

Powell, M., & Hemsley, D. R. (1984). Depression: A breakdown of perceptual defence. *British Journal of Psychology, 145,* 358–362.

Prince, M. (1910). *Subconscious phenomena* (Chap. 5, pp. 71–101). H. Münsterberg, T. Ribot, P. Janet, J. Jastrow, B. Hart, & M. Prince (Eds.). Boston, MA: Gorham.

Prince, M. (1921). *The unconscious: The fundamentals of human personality normal and abnormal* (2nd ed.). New York, NY: Macmillan.

Prince, M. (1925). Awareness, consciousness, co-consciousness and animal intelligence from the point of view of the data of abnormal psychology: A biological theory of consciousness. *Pedagogical Seminary, 32,* 166–188.

Prior, H., Schwarz, A., & Güntürkün, O. (2008). Mirror-induced behavior in the magpie (*Pica pica*): Evidence of self-recognition. *PLoS Biology, 6,* 1642–1650.

Proctor, H. C. (1991). The evolution of copulation in water mites: A comparative test for nonreversing characters. *Evolution, 45,* 558–567.

Ptito, M., Fumal, A., Schoenen, J., Gjedde, A., & Kupers, R. (2008). TMS of the occipital cortex induces tactile sensations in the fingers of blind Braille readers. *Experimental Brain Research, 184,* 193–200.

Pujol, R., & Lavigne-Rebillard, M. (1985). Early stage of innervation and sensory cell differentiation of the human fetal organ of Corti. *Acta Oto-Laryngolica, Suppl. 423,* 43–50.

Pylyshyn, Z. W. (1973). What the mind's eye tells the mind's brain: A critique of mental imagery. *Psychological Bulletin, 80,* 1–24.

Pylyshyn, Z. W. (1981). The imagery debate: Analogue media versus tacit knowledge. *Psychological Review, 88,* 16–45.

Pylyshyn, Z. W. (2003). Return of the mental image: Are there really pictures in the brain? *Trends in Cognitive Sciences, 7,* 113–118.

Raliou, M., Wiencis, A., Pillias, A.-M., Planchais, A., Eloit, C., Boucher, Y., et al. (2009). Nonsynonymous single nucleotide polymorphisms in human *tas1r1, tas1r3,* and mGluR1 and individual taste sensitivity to glutamate. *American Journal of Clinical Nutrition, 90,* 789S–799S.

Ramachandran, V. S., & Hirstein, W. (1998). The perception of phantom limbs. *Brain, 121,* 1603–1630.

Ramon y Cajal, S. (1888). Morfologia y conexiones de los elementos de la retina de las saves. *Revista Trimestral de Histología Normal y Patológica, 1,* 11–16.

Ramon y Cajal, S. (1889). Sur la morphologie et les connexions des elements de la rétine des oiseaux. *Anatomischer Anzeiger, 4,* 111–121.

Rasmussen, G. L. (1942). An efferent cochlear bundle. *Anatomical Record, 82,* 441.

Rasmussen, G. L. (1953). Further observations of the efferent cochlear bundle. *Journal of Comparative Neurology, 99,* 61–74.

Rattenborg, N. C. (2006). Evolution of slow-wave sleep and palliopallial connectivity in mammals and birds: A hypothesis. *Brain Research Bulletin, 69,* 20–29.

Rattenborg, N. C., Amlaner, C. J., & Lima, S. L. (2000). Behavioral, neurophysiological and evolutionary perspectives on unihemispheric sleep. *Neuroscience and Biobehavioral Reviews, 24,* 817–842.

Reber, A. S., & Allen, R. (1978). Analogy and abstraction strategies in synthetic grammar learning: A functionalist interpretation. *Cognition, 6,* 189–221.

Reber, A. S., & Allen, R. (2000). Individual differences in implicit learning: Implications for the evolution of consciousness. In R. G. Kunzendorf & B. Wallace (Eds.),

Individual differences in conscious experience (pp. 227–247). Amsterdam, The Netherlands: John Benjamins.

Reimer, A. A. (1971). Specificity of feeding chemoreceptors in Palythoa Psammophilia (Zoanthidea, Coelenterata). *Comparative and General Pharmacology, 2,* 383–396.

Reiner, A. (1986). Is prefrontal cortex found only in mammals? *Trends in Neurosciences, 9,* 298–300.

Reiner, A., & Karten, H. J. (1985). Comparison of olfactory bulb projections in pigeons and turtles. *Brain, Behavior and Evolution, 27,* 11–27.

Reiss, D., & Marino, L. (2001). Mirror self-recognition in the bottlenose dolphin: A case of cognitive convergence. *Proceedings of the National Academy of Sciences, 98,* 5937–5942.

Repérant, J., & Gallego, A. (1976). Fibres centrifuges dans la rétine humaine. *Archives d'Anatomie Microscopique et de Morphologie Expérimentale, 65,* 103–120.

Repérant, J., Miceli, D., Vesselkin, N. P., & Molotchnikoff, S. (1989). The centrifugal visual system of vertebrates: A century-old search reviewed. *International Review of Cytology, 118,* 115–171.

Repérant, J., Ward, R., Miceli, D., Rio, J. P., Médina, M., Kenigfest, N. B., & Vesselkin, N. P. (2006). The centrifugal visual system of vertebrates: A comparative analysis of its functional anatomical organization. *Brain Research Reviews, 52,* 1–57.

Ricciardi, E., Bonino, D., Sani, L., Vecchi, T., Guazzelli, M., Haxby, J. V., et al. (2009). Do we really need vision? How blind people "see" the actions of others. *Journal of Neuroscience, 29,* 9719–9724.

Richardson, A. (1977). The meaning and measurement of mental imagery. *British Journal of Psychology, 68,* 29–43.

Roberts, B. L., & Meredith, G. E. (1992). The efferent innervation of the ear: Variations on an enigma. In D. B. Webster, R. R. Fay, & A. N. Popper (Eds.), *The evolutionary biology of hearing* (pp. 185–210). New York, NY: Springer-Verlag.

Roberts, K. P., & Blades, M. (1995). Children's discrimination of memories for actual and pretend actions in a hiding task. *British Journal of Developmental Psychology, 13,* 321–333.

Robinson, C. J., Torebjörk, H. E., & LaMotte, R. H. (1983). Psychophysical detection and pain ratings of incremental thermal stimuli: A comparison with nociceptor responses in humans. *Brain Research, 274,* 87–106.

Roe, A. W., Pallas, S. L., Hahm, J.-O., & Sur, M. (1990). A map of visual space induced in primary auditory cortex. *Science, 250,* 818–820.

Rojas, L. M., McNeil, R., Cabana, T., & Lachapelle, P. (1999a). Behavioral, morphological and physiological correlates of diurnal and nocturnal vision in selected wading bird species. *Brain, Behavior, and Evolution, 53,* 227–242.

Rojas, L. M., McNeil, R., Cabana, T., & Lachapelle, P. (1999b). Diurnal and nocturnal visual capabilities in shorebirds as a function of their feeding strategies. *Brain, Behavior, and Evolution, 53,* 29–43.

Roopnarine, J. L., Hossain, Z., Gill, P., & Brophy, H. (1994). Play in the East Indian context. In J. L. Roopnarine, J. E. Johnson, & F. H. Hooper (Eds.), *Children's play in diverse cultures* (pp. 9–30). Albany, NY: State University of New York.

Ross, C. A., Miller, S. D., Reagor, P., Bjornson, L., Fraser, G. A., & Anderson, G. (1990). Schneiderian symptoms in multiple personality disorder and schizophrenia. *Comprehensive Psychiatry, 31,* 111–118.

Ross, C. A., Norton, G. R., & Wozney, K. (1989). Multiple personality disorder: Analysis of 326 cases. *Canadian Journal of Psychiatry, 34,* 413–418.

Rossetti, Z. L., & Carboni, S. (2005). Noradrenaline and dopamine elevations in the rat prefrontal cortex in spatial working memory. *Journal of Neuroscience, 25,* 2322–2329.

Roth, D. L., & Ingram, R. E. (1985). Factors in the self-deception questionnaire: Associations with depression. *Journal of Personality and Social Psychology, 48,* 243–251.

Ruseckaite, R., Lamb, T. D., Pianta, M. J., & Cameron, A. M. (2011). Human scotopic dark adaptation: Comparison of recoveries of psychophysical threshold and ERG b-wave sensitivity. *Journal of Vision, 11*(8), 1–16.

Ryou, J.-W., & Wilson, F. A. (2004). Making your next move: Dorsolateral prefrontal cortex and planning a sequence of actions in freely moving monkeys. *Cognitive, Affective & Behavioral Neuroscience, 4,* 430–443.

Sackeim, H. A. (1983). Self-deception, self-esteem, and depression: The adaptive value of lying to oneself. In J. Masling (Ed.), *Empirical studies of psychoanalytic theories* (Vol. 1, pp. 101–157). Hillsdale, NJ: Erlbaum.

Sacks, J. G., & Lindenberg, R. (1969). Efferent nerve fibers in the anterior visual pathways in bilateral congenital cystic eyeballs. *American Journal of Ophthalmology, 68,* 691–695.

Sakai, T., Kasuya, J., Kitamoto, T., & Aigaki, T. (2009). The *Drosophila* TRPA channel, Painless, regulates sexual receptivity in virgin females. *Genes, Brain and Behavior, 8,* 546–557.

Sass, L. A., & Parnass, J. (2003). Schizophrenia, consciousness, and the self. *Schizophrenia Bulletin, 29,* 427–444.

Satterlie, R. A., & Case, J. F. (1978). Neurobiology of the gorgonian coelenterates, Muricea californica and Lophogorgia chilensis. *Cell and Tissue Research, 187,* 379–396.

Savitz, J. B., van der Merwe, L., Newman, T. K., Solms, M., Stein, D. J., & Ramesar, R. S. (2008). The relationship between childhood abuse and dissociation: Is it influenced by catechol-O-methyltransferase (COMT) activity? *International Journal of Neuropsychopharmacology, 11,* 149–161.

Scates, K. W., Woods, C. I., & Azeredo, W. J. (1999). Inferior colliculus stimulation and changes in 2f1-f2 distortion product otoacoustic emissions in the rat. *Hearing Research, 128,* 51–60.

Schacter, D. L. (1989). On the relation between memory and consciousness: Dissociable interactions and conscious experience. In H. L. Roediger & F. I. M. Craik (Eds.), *Varieties of memory and consciousness: Essays in honour of Endel Tulving* (pp. 355–389). Hillsdale, NJ: Lawrence Erlbaum.

Scherer, K. R., & Wallbott, H. G. (1994). Evidence for universality and cultural variation of differential emotion response patterning. *Journal of Personality and Social Psychology, 66,* 310–328.

Schmelz, M. (2010). Itch and pain. *Neuroscience and Biobehavioral Reviews, 34,* 171–176.

Schmelz, M., Schmidt, R., Bickel, A., Handwerker, H. O., & Torebjörk, H. E. (Specific C-receptors for itch in human skin. *Journal of Neuroscience, 17,* 8003–8008.

Schmidt, R., Schmelz, M., Torebjörk, H. E., & Handwerker, H. O. (2000). Mechano-insensitive nociceptors encode pain evoked by tonic pressure to human skin. *Neuroscience, 98,* 793–800.

Schnapf, J. L., Kraft, T. W., & Baylor, D. A. (1987). Spectral sensitivity of human cone photoreceptors. *Nature, 325,* 439–441.

Schouenborg, J., Holmberg, H., & Wend, H. R. (1992). Functional organization of the nociceptive withdrawal reflexes. II. Changes of excitability and receptive fields after spinalization in the rat. *Experimental Brain Research, 90,* 469–478.

Schusterman, R. J., & Gisiner, R. (1988). Artificial language comprehension in dolphins and sea lions: The essential cognitive skills. *The Psychological Record, 38,* 311–348.

Schwab, I. R. (2012). *Evolution's witness: How eyes evolved.* Oxford, UK: Oxford University Press.

Scripture, E. W. (1895). Color sensitiveness. In E. W. Scripture (Ed.), *Thinking, feeling, doing* (pp. 170–179). Meadville, PA: Chautauqua Century.

Sedman, G. (1966). A comparative study of pseudohallucinations, imagery and true hallucinations. *British Journal of Psychiatry, 112,* 9–17.

Sheikh, A. A., & Kunzendorf, R. G. (1984). Imagery, physiology, and psychosomatic illness. *International Review of Mental Imagery, 1,* 95–138.

Sheikh, A. A., Kunzendorf, R. G., Sheikh, K. S., & Baer, S. M. (2003). Physiological consequences of imagery and related approaches. In A. A. Sheikh (Ed.), *Healing images: The role of imagination in health* (pp. 27–52). Amityville, NY: Baywood.

Sheikh, A. A., & Sheikh, K. S. (2003). Death imagery: Confronting death brings us to the threshold of life. In A. A. Sheikh (Ed.), *Healing images: The role of imagination in health* (pp. 471–488). Amityville, NY: Baywood.

Shepard, R. N. (1978). Externalization of mental images and the act of creation. In B. S. Randhawa & W. E. Coffman (Eds.), *Visual learning, thinking, and communication* (pp. 133–189). New York, NY: Academic.

Shepard, R. N. (1993). On the physical basis, linguistic representation, and conscious experience of colors. In G. Harman (Ed.), *Conceptions of the mind: Essays in honor of George A. Miller* (pp. 217–245). Hillsdale, NJ: Lawrence Erlbaum.

Shepard, R. N., & Cooper, L. A. (1992). Representation of colors in the blind, color-blind, and normally sighted. *Psychological Science, 3,* 97–104.

Sherman, S. M. (1974). Visual fields of cats with cortical and tectal lesions. *Science, 185,* 355–357.

Sherrington, C. S. (1911). *The integrative action of the nervous system.* New Haven, CT: Yale University Press.

Shewmon, D. A., Holmes, G. L., & Byrne, P. A. (1999). Consciousness in congenitally decorticate children: Developmental vegetative state as self-fulfilling prophecy. *Developmental Medicine and Child Neurology, 41,* 364–374.

Shukla, P., & Sinha, D. (1974). A developmental study of the relative efficacy of different pictorial cues in depth perception. *Indian Journal of Psychology, 49,* 220–230.

Siegel, J. M. (2008). Do all animals sleep? *Trends in Neurosciences, 31,* 208–213.

Siegel, J. M., Manger, P. R., Nienhuis, R., Fahringer, H. M., Shalita, T., & Pettigrew, J. D. (1999). Sleep in the platypus. *Neuroscience, 91,* 391–400.

Siegel, R. K. (1980). The psychology of life after death. *American Psychologist, 35,* 911–931.

Sierra, M., & Berrios, G. E. (2000). the Cambridge Depersonalization Scalr: A new instrument for the measurement of depersonalization. *Psychiatry Research, 93,* 153–164.

Sima, J. F., Schultheis, H., & Barkowsky, T. (2013). *Differences between spatial and visual mental representations. Frontiers in Psychology, 4*, article 240 (15 pages).

Singer, J. L. (1994). Imaginative play and adaptive development. In J. H. Goldstein (Ed.), *Toys, play, and child development* (pp. 6–26). New York, NY: Cambridge University Press.

Siniatchkin, M., Schlicke, C., & Stephani, U. (2011). Transcranial magnetic stimulation reveals high test-retest reliability phosphenes but not for suppression of visual perception. *Clinical Neurophysiology, 122,* 2475–2481.

Skavensky, A. A., Haddad, G., & Steinman, R. M. (1972). The extraretinal signal for the visual perception of direction. *Perception & Psychophysics, 11,* 287–290.

Skinner, B. F. (1974). *About behaviorism.* New York, NY: Alfred A. Knopf.

Smales, L. R., & Blankespoor, H. D. (1978). The epidermis and sensory organs of *Dugesia tigrina* (Turbellaria: Tricladida). *Cell and Tissue Research, 193,* 35–40.

Smart, J. J. C. (1959). Sensations and brain processes. *Philosophical Review, 68,* 141–156.

Smart, J. J. C. (1967). Religion and science. In P. Edwards (Ed.), *The encyclopedia of philosophy* (Vol. 7, pp. 158–163). New York, NY: Macmillan & Free Press.

Smith, E. S. J., & Lewin, G. R. (2009). Nociceptors: A phylogenetic view. *Journal of Comparative Physiology, 195,* 1089–1106.

Sneddon, L. U., Braithwaite, V. A., & Gentle, M. J. (2003). Do fish have nociceptors? Evidence for the evolution of a vertebrate sensory system. *Proceedings of the Royal Society: Section B. Biological Sciences, 270,* 1115–1121.

Soon, C. S., Brass, M., Heinze, H.-J., & Haynes, D.-J. (2008). Unconscious determinants of free decisions in the human brain. *Nature Neuroscience, 11,* 543–545.

Soon, C. S., He, A. H., Bode, S., & Haynes, D.-J. (2013). Predicting free choices for abstract intentions. *Proceedings of the National Academy of Sciences, 110,* 6217–6222.

Sperry, R. W. (1976). Mental phenomena as causal determinants in brain function. In G. Globus, G. Maxwell, & I. Savodnik (Eds.), *Consciousness and the brain* (pp. 161–177). New York, NY: Plenum.

Sperry, R. W., Zaidel, E., & Zaidel, D. (1979). Self recognition and social awareness in the deconnected minor hemisphere. *Neuropsychologia, 17,* 153–166.

Spetch, M. L., Rust, T. B., Kamil, A. C., & Jones, J. E. (2003). Searching by rules: Pigeons' (*Columba livia*) landmark-based search according to constant bearing or constant distance. *Journal of Comparative Psychology, 117,* 123–132.

Spiker, D., & Ricks, M. (1984). Visual self-recognition in autistic children: Developmental relationships. *Child Development, 55,* 214–225.

Spoendlin, H. (1966). *The organization of the cochlear receptor.* Basel, Switzerland: S. Karger.

Sprague, J. M. (1966). Interaction of cortex and superior colliculus in mediation of visually guided behavior in the cat. *Science, 153,* 1544–1547.

Starker, S. (1979). Fantasy in psychiatric patients: Exploring a myth. *Hospital & Community Psychiatry, 30,* 25–30.

Starker, S., & Jolin, A. (1983-1984). Occurrence and vividness of imagery in schizophrenic thought: A thought-sampling approach. *Imagination, Cognition and Personality, 3,* 49–60.

Stevens, S. S. (1961). To honor Fechner and repeal his law. *Science, 133,* 80–86.

Strange, B. A., Henson, R. N. A., Friston, K. J., & Dolan, R. J. (2001). Anterior prefrontal cortex mediates rule learning in humans. *Cerebral Cortex, 11,* 1040–1046.

Suarez, S. D., & Gallup, G. G., Jr. (1981). Self-recognition in chimpanzees and orangutans, but not gorillas. *Journal of Human Evolution, 10,* 175–188.

Suga, N., Xiao, Z., Ma, X., & Ji, W. (2002). Plasticity and corticofugal modulation for hearing in adult animals. *Neuron, 36,* 9–18.

Taylor, E. (1984). *William James on exceptional mental states: The 1896 Lowell lectures.* Amherst, MA: University of Massachusetts Press.

Tellegen, A., & Atkinson, G. (1974). Openness to absorbing and self-altering experiences ("absorption"), a trait related to hypnotic susceptibility. *Journal of Abnormal Psychology, 83,* 268–277.

Tellegen, A., Lykken, D. T., Bouchard, T. J., Wilcox, K. J., Segal, N. L., & Rich, S. (1988). Personality similarity in twins reared apart and together. *Journal of Personality and Social Psychology, 54,* 1031–1039.

Théoret, H., Merabet, L., & Pascual-Leone, A. (2004). Behavioral and neuroplastic changes in the blind: Evidence for functionally relevant cross-modal interactions. *Journal of Physiology, 98,* 221–233.

Titchener, E. B. (1909). *Lectures on the experimental psychology of the thought-processes.* New York, NY: Macmillan.

Torebjörk, H. E., LaMotte, R. H., & Robinson, C. J. (1984). Peripheral neural correlates of magnitude of cutaneous pain and hyperalgesia: Simultaneous recordings in humans of sensory judgments of pain and evoked responses in nociceptors with C-fibers. *Journal of Neurophysiology, 51,* 325–339.

Tracey, W. D., Wilson, R. I., Laurent, G., & Benzer, S. (2003). *painless*, a *Drosophila* gene essential for nociception. *Cell, 113,* 261–273.

Tsuno, Y., Kashiwadani, H., & Mori, K. (2008). Behavioral state regulation of dendrodendritic synaptic inhibition in the olfactory bulb. *Journal of Neuroscience, 28,* 9227–9238.

Untermeyer, L. (1951). *The road not taken: An introduction to Robert Frost.* New York, NY: Henry Holt.

Vaughan, C. J. (1966). The development and use of an operant technique to provide evidence for visual imagery in the rhesus monkey under "sensory deprivation." *Dissertation Abstracts, 26,* 6191.

Venneri, A., Pentore, R., Cobelli, M., Nichelli, P., & Shanks, M. F. (2012). Translocation of the embodied self without visuospatial neglect. *Neuropsychologia, 50,* 973–978.

Ventura, J., & Mathieu, M. (1959). Exogenous fibres of the retina. *Transactions of the Canadian Ophthalmological Society, 22,* 184–196.

Ventura, J., & Mathieu, M. (1960). Silver impregnation of whole retinas. *A.M.A. Archives of Ophthalmology, 64,* 528–535.

Veuillet, E., Magna, A., Ecalle, J., Thai-Van, H., & Collet, L. (2007). Auditory processing disorder in children with reading disabilities: Effect of audiovisual training. *Brain, 130,* 2915–2928.

von Helmholtz, H. (1962). *Treatise on physiological optics* (Vol. III; J. P. C. Southall, Ed.). Mineola, NY: Dover. (Original work published 1910 in German)

Voss, J. J. (1978). Colorimetric and photometric properties of a 2° fundamental observer. *Color Research and Application, 3,* 125–128.

Voss, M. (2000). Neurophysiological and behavioral responses to olfactory stimuli in the snail Helix pomatia L. *Physiological Research/Academia Scientiarum Bohemoslovaca, 49,* 463–469.

Wallace, B., & Kokoszka, A. (1995). Fluctuations in hypnotic susceptibility and imaging ability over a 16-hour period. *International Journal of Clinical and Experimental Hypnosis, 43,* 20–33.

Walters, E. T. (2009). Chronic pain, memory, and injury: Evolutionary clues from snail and rat nociceptors. *International Journal of Comparative Psychology, 22,* 127–140.

Wang, D. Y.-C., Kumar, S., & Hedges, S. B. (1999). Divergence time estimates for the early history of animal phyla and the origin of plants, animals and fungi. *Proceedings of the Royal Society: B. Biological Sciences, 266,* 163–171.

Washburn, M. F., & Bentley, I. M. (1906). The establishment of an association involving color-discrimination in the creek chub, Semotilus atromaculatus. *Journal of Comparative Neurology & Psychology, 16,* 113–125.

Watanabe, S. (2002). Preference for mirror images and video image in Java sparrows (Padda oryzivora). *Behavioural Processes, 60,* 35–39.

Watson, J. B. (1913). Image and affection in behavior. *Journal of Philosophy, Psychology, and Scientific Methods, 10,* 421–428.

Watson, N. A., & Rohde, K. (1994). Two new sensory receptors in Gyrodactylus sp. (Platyhelminthes, Monogenea, Monopisthocotylea). *Parasitology Research, 80,* 442–445.

Wegner, D. M. (2002). *The illusion of conscious will.* Cambridge, MA: MIT Press.

Wegner, D. M. (2003). The mind's best trick: How we experience conscious will. *Trends in Cognitive Sciences, 7,* 65–69.

Wegner, D. M. (2004). Précis of *The illusion of conscious will. Behavioral and Brain Sciences, 27,* 649–692.

Weiskrantz, L. (2002). Prime-sight and blindsight. *Consciousness and Cognition, 11,* 568–581.

Weiss, O., & Meyer, D. L. (1988). Odor stimuli modulate retinal excitability in fish. *Neuroscience Letters, 93,* 209–213.

Welch-Ross, M. K. (1995). Developmental changes in preschoolers' ability to distinguish between memories of performed, pretended, and imagined actions. *Child Development, 10,* 421–441.

Wild, J. M., Krützfeldt, N. O. E., & Kubke, M. F. (2010). Connections of the auditory brainstem in a songbird, *Taeniopygia guttata.* III. Projections of the superior olive and lateral lemniscal nuclei. *Journal of Comparative Neurology, 518,* 2149–2167.

Wilkinson, C., & Hyman, I. A., Jr. (1998). Individual differences related to two types of memory errors: Word lists may not generalize to autobiographical memory. *Applied Cognitive Psychology, 12,* S29–S46.

Williams, H. (1989). Multiple representations and auditory-motor interactions in the avian song system. *Annals of the New York Academy of Sciences, 563,* 148–164.

Willner, P. (1978). What does the headless cockroach remember? *Animal Learning & Behavior, 6,* 249–257.

Winograd, E., Peluso, J. P., & Glover, T. A. (1998). Individual differences in susceptibility to memory illusions. *Applied Cognitive Psychology, 12,* S5–S27.

Wolter, J. R. (1960). Regenerative potentialities of the centrifugal fibers of the human optic nerve. *Archives of Ophthalmology, 64,* 697–707.

Wolter, J. R. (1965a). The centrifugal nerves in the human optic tract, chiasm, optic nerve, and retina. *Transactions of the American Ophthalmological Society, 63,* 678–707.

Wolter, J. R. (1965b). The reactions of the centrifugal nerves of the human eye: After photocoagulation, occlusion of the central retinal artery and bilateral enucleation. In J. W. Rohen (Ed.), *The structure of the eye* (pp. 85–95). Stuttgart, Germany: F. K. Schattauer-Verlag.

Wolter, J. R. (1979). Electron microscopic demonstration of centrifugal nerve fibers in the human optic nerve. *Gräfes Archiv für klinische und experimentelle Ophthalmologie, 210,* 31–41.

Wolter, J. R. (1991). Reaction of centrifugal nerves in perforated peripheral retina. *Neuro-ophthalmology, 11,* 189–193.

Wolter, J. R., & Knoblich, R. R. (1965). Pathway of centrifugal fibres in the human optic nerve, chiasm, and tract. *British Journal of Ophthalmology, 49,* 246–250.

Wood, B. D., & Bell, J. C. (1920). Solution of problems in geometry. *Journal of Educational Psychology, 11,* 316–326.

Wright, K. A. (1977). Labial sense organs of the nematode, Heterakis gallinarum. *Journal of Parasitology, 63,* 528–539.

Wundt, W. (1894). *Lectures on human and animal psychology* (J. E. Creighton & E. B. Titchener, Trans.). New York, NY: Macmillan. (Original work published 1863 in German)

Wyman, E., Rakoczy, H., & Tomasello, M. (2009). Young children understand multiple pretend identities in their object play. *British Journal of Developmental Psychology, 27,* 385–404.

Xiao, Z., & Suga, N. (2002). Modulation of cochlear hair cells by the auditory cortex in the mustached bat. *Nature Neuroscience, 5,* 57–63.

Xu, S. Y., Cang, C. L., Liu, X. F., Peng, Y. Q., Ye, Y. Z., Zhao, Z. Q., & Guo, A. K. (2006). Thermal nociception in adult *Drosophila*: Behavioral characterization and the role of the *painless* gene. *Genes, Brain and Behavior, 5,* 602–613.

Yager, D. D. (1999). Structure, development, and evolution of insect auditory systems. *Microscopy Research and Technique, 47,* 380–400.

Yoshioka, K., Tanahasi, M., & Uchida, W. (2010). Behavioral and urological evaluation of a testicular pain model. *Urology, 75,* 943–948.

Zarroung, E. A. (1975). The frequency of visual hallucinations in schizophrenic patients in Saudi Arabia. *British Journal of Psychiatry, 127,* 553–555.

Zeki, S. (2001). Localization and globalization in conscious vision. *Annual Review of Neuroscience, 24,* 57–86.

Zeman, A. Z. J., Della Sala, S., Torrens, L. A., Gountouna, V.-E., McGonigle, D. J., & Logie, R. H. (2010). Loss of imagery phenomenology with intact visuo-spatial task performance: A case of "blind imagination." *Neuropsychologia, 48,* 145–155.

Zhong, L. (2012). Neuronal and molecular basis of nociception and thermosensation in Drosophila melanogaster. *Dissertation Abstracts International: Section B. The Sciences and Engineering, 72,* 3872.

Zung, W. W., & Gianturco, J. A. (1971). Personality dimension and the self-rating depression scale. *Journal of Clinical Psychology 27,* 247–248.

Index